Health Hints for Hikers

SANDI DALE

Health Hints for Hikers

Albert P. Rosen, M.D.

published by the
NEW YORK-NEW JERSEY
TRAIL CONFERENCE

New York 1994

The New York-New Jersey Trail Conference wishes to acknowledge the help of The Lucius N. Littauer Foundation in the publication of this book.

Library of Congress Cataloging-in-Publication Data

Rosen, Albert P.
    Health hints for hikers / by Albert P. Rosen.
       p.   cm.
    Includes indexes.
    ISBN 1-880775-02-6
    1. Hiking—Health aspects. 2. Hiking injuries.   I. New York-New Jersey Trail Conference. II. Title.
RC1220.M6R67   1994
612.6—dc20   94-31690
                                           CIP

Cover design by Steve Butfilowski

Page design by Alice L. Tufel

CONTENTS

EDITOR'S PREFACE

Dr. Albert Rosen has been writing the "Health Hints" column for the *Trail Walker* (the official publication of the New York-New Jersey Trail Conference) "since time immemorial," as he puts it. Over the years, his clear and practical advice, his emphasis on prevention, and his delightful sense of humor have endeared him to thousands of readers, who have come to think of him as their very own family doctor.

Dr. Rosen's readers have often asked that old columns be rerun, and many readers have inquired whether any compilation of the "Health Hints" columns is available—and that is how this book came into being. So many people expressed an interest in having a collection of the good doctor's advice columns that we asked him if he'd like to put one together. In the end, we were able to complete this project thanks to generous help from The Lucius N. Littauer Foundation, to whom we are most grateful.

This little volume, then, represents Dr. Rosen's answers to hikers' most frequently asked questions over the years. The original "Health Hints" columns, which appeared in a question-and-answer format in the *Trail Walker*, have been updated, edited, and organized into a structure that will be helpful for hikers who want no-nonsense medical advice on common problems associated with the trail. This collection is not meant to be exhaustive or to substitute for actual medical attention when it is needed—but it will be invaluable for anyone who wants to be able to administer emergency self-help on the trail, to overcome aches and pains that could ruin or prevent a hike, and to recognize the symptoms of common hiking-related medical problems and be able to treat those problems. What's more, Dr. Rosen's warm, witty, and down-to-earth style makes for pleasurable reading even if you're not looking for advice on a specific ailment.

Other guides may offer medical and first-aid guidance to hikers, but this book is unique because of its author: Readers wanted a guide *by Dr. Rosen*. The loyal following that he has deservedly built over the years demanded that this book be published. With its availability, we hope that other hikers, as well as old fans, will benefit from and enjoy the mixture of helpful advice, whimsy, and wisdom that are on these pages.

Happy trails!

Alice L. Tufel
Editor

ACKNOWLEDGMENTS

I want to express my gratitude to the Trail Conference and to its Publication Chairman, Daniel D. Chazin, for their efforts in taking dozens of "Health Hints" columns, which appeared in the *Trail Walker* for many, many years, and putting them into book form.

I especially want to thank Alice L. Tufel, the present editor of the *Trail Walker* and of this book, for making order out of chaos, which was a herculean task. Just deciphering my notes makes her a wonder woman.

I am indebted to Joachim Oppenheimer, a physician, scholar, and hiker, who reviewed the manuscript and made many valuable suggestions, as did my son, Jonathan Rosen, an ardent mountaineer with a special interest in high-altitude medicine. Thanks also to Drs. John C. Hall and John M. Dunn for reviewing the manuscript and making some good suggestions.

This book would never have happened without the help of Frances (Fran) Gass, who has worked with me for over twenty years as office manager, typist, sounding board—a woman with marvelous mechanical talents as well as a fellow bread-maker.

Finally, I want to express my gratitude to Claudia Allocco, the librarian at the Valley Hospital, and her staff, who spent countless hours gathering articles for me.

Albert P. Rosen

CHAPTER ONE
Coping with Discomfort on the Trail

Various kinds of health problems can affect our enjoyment of hiking. They include minor and not-so-minor injuries that occur on the trail, serious accidents and life-threatening emergencies, and general aches and pains. For all of them, knowledge of first aid and self-help techniques can make the difference between comfort and discomfort, and may even save a life.

First Aid and Self-Help

Hiking accidents usually occur in areas where doctors and health facilities are not readily available. Therefore, it behooves hikers to be capable of rendering first aid to themselves and to others. It would be ideal if all hike leaders had the capability of administering first aid, including cardiopulmonary resuscitation.

Every hiker should have a **first-aid kit** in his or her pack. Prepared kits can be purchased in drug stores, surgical supply stores, and camping equipment stores. However, I think it is a better idea to make your own kit and tailor it to meet your needs. Keep in mind that the more expensive the kit, the bulkier and heavier it becomes. The ideal kit is small, compact, and water-proof.

The first-aid kit should contain adhesive tape, sterile gauze pads, alcohol preps, clear tape, Band-Aids®, Telfa® sterile pads, antihistamines, aspirin, safety pins, and Moleskin® (or Molefoam®, which some people prefer). Optional items include a triangular bandage (or a large kerchief or bandanna), surgical bandages such as an Ace® bandage, and Second Skin®, made by Spenco. Duct tape has many uses, too; it can be used to prevent a "hot spot" from becoming a full-blown blister and to immobilize fractures. It might be wise to keep a pair of latex gloves for use when dealing with bleeding wounds. If you are prone to "downhill knees" (sore joints), you can use an Ace® bandage to immobilize your knee before starting out. An Ace® bandage is also excellent for wrapping around the site of a snake bite if it is on an extremity, and for wrapping around a splint when immobilizing a fracture. Forceps are useful for removing ticks and splinters.

The clear tape, which comes in various sizes, is useful for bringing wound edges together in case of a laceration. One of its advantages is that the wound can be seen, so you know the edges are together. (Dermiclear®, made by Johnson & Johnson, and Transpore®, made by 3M, are good clear tapes; or use a generic brand—which may be less expensive—if you can find one.)

The safety pins are useful to pin a sleeve against the chest so an upper extremity can be immobilized. The triangular bandage or large kerchief, fashioned into a sling, can serve the same purpose.

The Moleskin® is invaluable for protecting blisters before they become painful.

The aspirin has multiple uses. It is an adequate, safe pain reliever, and can be used for headaches, muscle pains, joint pains, and toothaches. It is not as effective as a narcotic, but it is safer, cheaper, and readily available—and your chance of being arrested for possession of narcotics is eliminated. Aspirin also helps control fever. The usual dose, two tablets (325 milligrams or five grains per tablet) every four hours, is relatively safe unless you have an allergy to aspirin.

Aspirin does prolong bleeding time for four to seven days after ingestion. However, that usually is no problem. Medical studies have shown that aspirin taken on an ongoing basis reduces the incidence of heart attack, but consult your doctor before you start. There is usually no need for brand-name enteric-coated aspirin or buffered aspirin; if taken with food, you shouldn't have any problem. If you do have problems, try buffered or enteric aspirin.[1]

If you have a problem with aspirin, use acetaminophen, which reduces pain and fever, or ibuprofen, which is anti-inflammatory as well; both are available over the counter. Ibuprofen should be taken with food. The usual dose for acetaminophen is 325 milligrams, and for ibuprofen it is 400 milligrams (two 200-milligram tablets), every four to six hours. For alleviating more severe pain, two 500-milligram acetaminophen capsules are very effective.

Telfa® pads are good because you can place them over an injured area and they won't adhere to the raw wound.

In addition to their ''itch-suppressing'' properties, antihistamines have several uses, which include counteracting the effects of insect bites, relieving a stuffy nose, and providing a general anti-allergy action.

---

[1]Enteric aspirin is specially treated to pass through the stomach unaltered and disintegrate in the intestines, thus circumventing stomach problems.

If you or your doctor have no special favorite, I suggest you get Chlortrimeton® tablets (4 milligrams), which can be purchased over-the-counter, eliminating the expense and hassle of obtaining a prescription. One of its side effects is drowsiness, so don't drive after taking it. It comes in handy, however, if you have trouble sleeping on the hard ground or in a noisy shelter. The usual dose for Chlortrimeton® is one tablet every six to eight hours. Benadryl® (25 milligrams) also can be purchased over-the-counter and has a similar action. It is excellent to take at night if you have an allergic nose.

If you have a known allergy to insect stings, your doctor can provide adrenaline (trade name, Adrenalin®) and a syringe—this treatment is only for life-threatening reactions, not for localized swelling. *(See Insect Bites and Stings, page 63.)*

Emergency Life-Saving Techniques

Anywhere, any time, and any place, someone may stop breathing and show no pulse—and you might be there. What do you do? Immediately initiate **cardiopulmonary resuscitation** (CPR) and save a life.

CPR maintains breathing and blood circulation until further help can be obtained or until the body resumes these functions on its own. It must be applied within four minutes to prevent irreversible brain damage, and it is useful for victims of heart attack, accidental electrocution, near-drowning, drug overdose, choking, or smoke inhalation.

Heart attack is the most common cause of sudden death. Everyone should know its early signs so proper medical attention can be obtained. Uncomfortable pressure, squeezing fullness or pain in the center of the chest behind the breastbone, sweating, nausea, shortness of breath, and weakness are all indicative of a potential heart attack. These signs may subside, but they can return. If breathing stops, that is the time to apply CPR. CPR can also be used if someone stops breathing because of choking—but an airway must be established first. *Do not give CPR until you remove airway obstructions*.

Anyone who is choking because of a foreign body, such as food, stuck in the airway, should be given the **Heimlich maneuver** *unless* he or she can speak in a normal voice and is capable of coughing, in which case the Heimlich maneuver should *not* be used. You should also do a finger sweep of the mouth to make certain there is no foreign body in the posterior pharynx. To use the Heimlich maneuver, put the heel of your palm on the victim's upper abdominal area, below the sternum (breastbone), and place your other hand over it. Give a firm thrust upward—do this six to ten times. If the patient is conscious and coughing, *do* *not* undertake this maneuver. Give the body a chance to handle the problem itself.

According to *CPR*, a leaflet put out by the American Heart Association, the three things that have to be remembered to initiate cardiopulmonary resuscitation are simple as A-B-C: Airway, Breathing, and Circulation.

Airway. If the person is unconscious, open the airway. The victim should be flat on his or her back. If you must roll the victim over, move the entire body as a total unit. Lift the neck up gently with one hand—assuming there is no evidence of a neck injury. Use the other hand on the forehead so the forehead is low and the chin is high—this opens the airway. Then place your ear close to the victim's mouth and listen for breathing sounds. Try to feel breath on your cheek. Look for chest and stomach movement. If none of these signs is present, the victim is not breathing.

Breathing. The best way to provide rescue breathing is to use mouth-to-mouth resuscitation. The technique is as follows: While maintaining the head tilt you used to open the airway, check the mouth for foreign objects that can get stuck in the windpipe, such as chewing gum. If you find something, remove it. Pinch the victim's nose shut, with the chin still pointing up. Immediately give two slow breaths (1½ to 2 seconds per breath) by placing your mouth over the victim's mouth.[1] Watch the chest rise and allow for exhalation between breaths.

Circulation. Check for a pulse by locating the carotid artery, in the groove beside the voice box. If there is no pulse, you must provide artificial circulation in addition to rescue breathing. Locate your own carotid artery using your index and middle fingers. Do it enough times that you can easily find it.

Artificial circulation is provided by means of external cardiac compression, which forces the heart to pump blood. To perform external cardiac compression, kneel at the victim's side near the chest. Locate the lowest part of the sternum (breastbone) and place the heel of one hand about one inch above that point. Depress the sternum two inches, then relax. This maneuver is easier to do if you place one hand on top of the other. Keep your hands in position between compressions. If you are alone with the victim, you must provide both mouth-to-mouth resuscitation and cardiac compression. The ratio for anyone eight years or older is fifteen chest compressions to two quick breaths, and the rate is eighty compressions per minute. If there are two rescuers, a breath is given after every fifth compression, and the rate is sixty compres-

---

[1]Until recently, four quick breaths were recommended.

sions per minute. For victims younger than eight years, the rate should be 100 compressions per minute, with a compression–breath ratio of 5:1.

CPR is best learned with supervised instruction. Ask your chapter of the American Heart Association or the American Red Cross for more information about CPR training.

It's good to learn the symptoms of heart attack and the procedure for administering CPR. CPR in the backwoods is a challenge, but it should be tried and it should be continued until the rescuers become exhausted. It's good for your families and close friends to know heart attack symptoms and CPR, too. The life they save may be their own . . . or yours.

Responding to Accidents and Injuries

Because professional medical services are not available on the trail, hikers should familiarize themselves with the proper techniques for examining and caring for an accident victim until definite medical help can be secured. If possible, hikers should avail themselves of the first-aid courses given by the American Red Cross.

The severity of the problem is usually self-evident. It does not require a medical genius to recognize loss of consciousness, stoppage of breathing, or severe bleeding. The latter two require immediate action, as time is of the utmost importance if certain death is to be avoided. The most experi-enced member of the group should decide whether a vic-tim can be evacuated under his or her own power. If there is any doubt, carry the victim out, assuming you have enough people. If evac-uation is not possible, keep the victim warm and reas-sured, and send for help.

> *It does not require a medical genius to recognize loss of consciousness, stoppage of breathing, or severe bleeding.*

If you tend to be acci-dent-prone, get yourself a good health and accident policy. If you feel you are a lost cause, get a life insurance policy.

Fractures and Sprains

Fractures and sprains are bad news no matter where or when they happen, but the problem is magnified when it occurs in the typical hiking locale, which is usually not near medical facilities. Fractures are particularly problematic, and some are worse than others. **Sprains** and **simple fractures**, which have no open wound and no marked deformity (other than some possible swell-ing), are more manageable than **compound fractures**, which have an open wound extending from the fracture site to the skin. All sprains and fractures should be immobilized, and ice should be applied if it is available.

A hiker who suffers a fracture above the pelvis can be walked out of the hiking area, assuming he or she is conscious and the neck is unharmed.

A hiker who experiences a lower-extremity fracture, however, is generally precluded from walking out to get medical help, and usually has to be littered out of the hiking area. If the victim is hiking with at least four people, the other hikers might be able to carry out the victim themselves. A litter can be made of parkas or ponchos and saplings. Otherwise, a member of the group has to go out and bring help in.

Other situations that call for a litter include skull fractures (with the accompanying loss of consciousness), shock, or possible fractures of the neck and back. Shock is manifested by a weak pulse, dilated pupils, nausea, and pale, cold, moist skin. Hikers who are in shock should be kept flat unless they are having difficulty breathing; in that case, the victim's head should be elevated. A shock victim should be kept warm and encouraged to drink as much fluid as possible (assuming there is no loss of consciousness and the person is capable of swallowing).

The area of any fracture or suspected fracture

should be immobilized, as should the joints on either side of the fracture site. Tenderness, pain, and sometimes an open wound identify the fracture site. Fractures can be immobilized with triangular bandages, adhesive tape, or belts. Ice axes, walking sticks, or saplings can be used as splints, held in place with cord, belts, or surgical bandages. I know one leader, Ted Billings of Paragon Guides, who uses a ski pole as a walking stick, on which he wraps a batch of duct tape. He uses this tape to immobilize fractures as well as to repair boots, fix holes in tents, and cover blisters. The pole itself can be used as a splint. Triangular bandages can be made into a sling for upper-extremity fractures and used for immobilizing a clavicle fracture with a figure-eight application. Open wounds should be treated with antiseptic and sterile gauze dressing.

Lightweight splints, such as Sam splints, which can be used to immobilize fractures, are now available. They are especially handy above treeline or in areas where no saplings are available to make a temporary splint. With a few lightweight splints and a few Ace® bandages, a group is much better prepared to immobilize fractures.

There are some things you can do to try to avoid fractures. Don't walk on ice unless you have crampons. Be leery of moss, lichen, wet leaves, and wet rocks, which are deceptively slippery. Watch where you put your feet when gabbing with a fellow hiker. Step *over* logs, not on them, as wet logs are treacherous. Use a walking stick or Alpenstock, an ice axe, or a ski pole (or two), so you have more than one point of contact with the ground. (This is especially helpful for people with poor balance.) It seems to me that hikers in Europe use walking sticks far more than we do in the States. In fact, a great many of them use umbrellas (which also come in handy when it rains).

Sometimes, no matter how careful you are, you can still suffer a sprain or fracture. If you do, follow the advice above, and remember that you will recover.

Injured Skin

Common skin problems on a hike or backpack trip are cuts, abrasions, and lacerations. They are best treated by gently washing them with soap and rinsing with running water. If running water is not available, use the water in a water bottle or canteen. Make certain you remove all foreign particles, and apply a bandage for protection against further contamination.

If neither soap nor water is available, use isopropyl alcohol (rubbing alcohol). Hydrogen peroxide is a poor antiseptic, but the frothy action is an aid in cleaning wounds. Tincture of iodine, which stings, and Betadine®, which does not, are fairly effective. The use of an over-the-counter antibiotic ointment such as Neosporin® or bacitracin is questionable, since it may cause allergic reactions and growth of resistant organisms. Betadine®, zephiran chloride, and Hibiclens are all acceptable antiseptics.

If none of these is available, don't fret. Injured skin, even if left alone, has superb recuperative powers. Moreover, bacteria on the skin surface are harmless. The majority of organisms that enter a wound are handled by the body's immune system and not by the germicide applied.

Lacerations in which the skin edges are separated should be pulled together by butterfly bandages. Even better is clear tape, which enables you to see the condition of the wound at all times. If the wound bleeds excessively, use firm pressure on it until the bleeding stops; don't just dab at it.

There is rarely a need for a tourniquet. Direct pressure is the best method to stop bleeding, and a tourniquet should be used only as a last resort, if direct pressure does not work. A tourniquet left on too long can cause more damage than the wound.

Burns from Fire

I don't usually associate burns with outdoor activities but they occasionally do occur in the outdoors. At some time we've suffered burns from touching a hot stove, a campfire, or a hot pot. Many of the synthetic garments, such as polypropylene, can melt with sustained high heat and cause skin burns. These types of burns usually involve a very small area, and all they require are cold applications at the time of the accident, using cold water or ice, if available. Then apply whatever ointment you have, such as first-aid cream or an antibiotic ointment, followed by a dressing, if necessary. If the burn is more extensive, the treatment is the same, but when you return home you should find out whether you have had a tetanus immunization within the past ten years. (If you have not, you should get one, regardless of whether you've been burned.)

> *Take care of your skin. It has to last you a lifetime.*

In cases of third-degree burns, the entire depth of the skin is destroyed, including the subcutaneous tissue, and the pain is extremely severe. Do not try to treat this type of burn on the trail or in camp; find the nearest medical facility as soon as possible. Do the same for any extensive burn, regardless of the degree. Severe burns are true medical emergencies.

There is no place in the treatment of burns for lard, grease, butter, oil, vitamin E, and over-the-counter burn ointments. As for aloe vera, I feel it is as effective in treating burns as garlic is in warding off vampires.

Take care of your skin. It has to last you a lifetime.

Eye Injuries

Hiking can be dangerous to your eyes. Those of us who have been hit in the face by snapping branches can vouch for it. For eye emergencies, use the following items from your first-aid kit: sterile gauze pads (2" x 2") and adhesive tape. The sterile gauze pads can be used as eye patches, kept in place with adhesive tape. If you are going on a trip of several days duration in an area where medical help is not available, consider carrying eye ointments or drops in your first-aid kit, but get medical guidance for obtaining and using the preparations. In snow and strong sun conditions, wear sunglasses to avoid snow blindness, which can be extremely painful.

A common complaint is "I have something in my eye," accompanied by intense discomfort. For relief, a companion can remove the offending particle. If it is not seen on the eye or by pulling down the lower lid, look under the upper lid. Do this by using a toothpick, a matchstick, or a twig as a fulcrum across the upper part of the lid. Grab the margin of the lid and fold it upward over the fulcrum; the speck will be visible. Remove it with the tip of a tissue, a handkerchief, or a wisp of cotton.

If the foreign body is on the cornea and it doesn't budge with the first try, patch the eye and get medical help on the way home.

Conjunctivitis, or "pink eye," is manifested by inflammation and pus. The eyelids may be stuck together. Wash the eye with water, and place a pea-sized amount of antibiotic ointment inside the lower lid, or one drop of medication (prescription required) in liquid form every four hours when needed. Apply the ointment every three to four hours. This situation is not an emergency and many times clears itself in short order, so finish your trip. However, conjunctivitis is very contagious upon contact, so don't share your towel or washcloth with anyone, and keep your fingers out of your eyes. If it hasn't cleared up by the time you get home, see your doctor.

Sudden burning or itching in an eye is usually caused by an allergen, such as pollen. Wash the eye with water, using the cap of a water bottle as an eye cup. That may wash out the irritant. Photophobia, or an abnormal intolerance of light, coupled with pain, indicates damage to the cornea. If the pain is intolerable, get medical help as soon as possible. If you are fairly comfortable, however, you can finish your hike. Patch the eye, and have it checked at a medical facility when you return home.

If your vision is impaired and you have the sensation of seeing through a film of water, the outer layer of the eye may have been damaged. Patch the eye and get help at the earliest convenience. If you are not experiencing any marked discomfort, you can keep hiking. If there is a loss of vision or bleeding from the eye associated with trauma, patch the eye, do not apply any medications, and get to the nearest emergency room or eye doctor as fast as possible.

Small lid lacerations are not serious as long as they do not involve the lid margin. Sometimes they can be closed with a small strip of tape. Lacerations involving the lid margins or the tissue next to the bridge of the nose that covers the lachrymal duct require the help of an eye doctor.

Vomiting and nausea associated with a painful eye may be caused by glaucoma. Get help fast.

Avoid getting chemicals such as bug repellent in your eyes. Pyrinate A-200® is excellent for head lice but causes corneal ulcerations and can ruin an outing.

Aches and Pains

So you're not feeling that great, but you still want to go hiking? Or you're on the trail, and an old pain or problem acts up? You don't have to postpone your hike or turn back! You can take some simple steps to prevent or minimize discomfort on the trail so you can keep on hiking safely and comfortably.

Problems with Feet

Feet are the Achilles heel of the hiker, and the first line of defense is a pair of well-fitting boots. The following guide may provide a proper fit.

Try on boots with the type of socks you plan to wear with them. With the boots unlaced, and the toes touching the front, you should be able to place a finger between your heel and the back of the boot; with the boot tightly laced, your heel should not lift up more than an eighth of an inch from the heel cup. To make certain that your toes do not jam against the front of the boot, which occurs on descending, try tapping the floor with your toe or stand on a steep incline. The toes should not hit the front of the boot. Remember: If the boots don't feel comfortable in the store, they won't feel comfortable on the trail, either.

Boots should not be broken in on a hike. The procedure I follow is to wear new footgear in my office. As soon as they cause any discomfort, I put on my usual footgear for the remainder of the day. I do this daily until I can wear my new boots all day without discomfort.

The next step is to take a short hike with the boots and get them wet by walking in a small stream, and continue walking with them until they dry out. Some of the newer boots made of Gore-Tex® and canvas do not require the wetting process, but it is effective with leather boots. Several manufacturers are offering hiking shoes that are offsprings of their running shoes. They are lighter and more comfortable but less rugged.

Wear two pairs of socks so the shearing action is between socks rather than between skin and socks. The sock next to the skin can be light wool, polypropylene, or any of the other synthetics that have a wicking action. The outer sock should be heavy wool, such as a Ragg sock, or a thick synthetic such as polypropylene. Make certain that the socks fit, and eliminate any folds or lumps.

Keep your toenails short and cut straight across to prevent ingrown nails. If you have ingrown toenails, get professional help before you hit the trail.

These suggestions should prevent, or at least cut down on, blisters—a leading cause of painful feet.

Blisters
To prevent a blister from forming, don't keep walking when you feel a "hot spot"—stop immediately and cover the area with Moleskin® or duct tape. If neither one is available, use an adhesive bandage. If your feet perspire excessively, use a drying powder such as Zeasorb® or corn starch. Once a blister has formed, don't cut it. If it isn't too large, leave it alone. Puncture a large blister at the outer edge with a sterlized needle. The fluid will drain through the puncture hole.

After puncturing, cover the blister with a gauze pad or a Telfa® pad, and apply Moleskin® over the pad and the blister. This will protect the surface of the blister. If the roof is torn off, apply flexible collodion or tincture of benzoin if either is available; if not, apply an antibiotic ointment, cover with gauze or a Telfa® pad, and then apply Moleskin®.

A fellow hiker, Ken Lloyd, sent me an excerpt from the *Walking Journal* on the treatment of blisters, submitted by Dr. Howard Palamarchuk. He uses Second Skin®, a plastic gel material impregnated with a large amount of water, which cushions, soothes, and protects the blister. Second Skin® comes in sheets in a packet. Cut out a piece large enough to cover the blister and tape it on. Dr. Palamarchuk recommends Micropore® paper tape. Then tape a pad over it, to keep the Second Skin® from sliding around. Using Second Skin® allows you to keep going while the blister heals.

Calluses, Corns, and Warts

Calluses, usually protective, can become large enough to be troublesome. If they are painful, soak them in warm, soapy water for fifteen minutes and then rub with a pumice stone. **Corns** can be treated with plasters or Mediplast® pads. **Warts** are caused by a virus. They frequently go away without treatment. If they are bothersome, and they do not respond to standard over-the-counter treatments (such as Compound W®), they can be excised, cauterized, or laser-treated by a physician.

Plantar warts can be treated with Mediplast® pads or Compound W®. If Compound W® does not work, try 40 percent salicylic acid pads—cut a piece that just covers the wart and keep it in place with adhesive tape. Replace the pad when it falls off.

Toe Jamming

Toe jamming is usually caused by boots that were not fitted properly (see page 19). However, if you are stuck with a set of foot gear that is associated with toe jamming, get some Dr. Scholl's® adhesive foam, cut out a piece to fit the forward part of the shoe, and press it down so it adheres. That should help prevent the toes from slipping forward. Tightening your boot laces may eliminate or lessen the toe jamming. If these methods fail, you can hike either on level trails, or on trails that only ascend.

Skin Problems

Dry, cracking skin on your feet can also cause problems. This condition is aggravated by poor circulation and cold weather, with its accompanying "frozen feet." There are times when the superficial skin comes off in layers and deep cracks develop. Skin moisturizers such as Eucerin®, Aveeno®, and petroleum jelly (Vaseline®) are helpful and are relatively inexpensive if purchased in pound jars. Apply after soaking feet in warm water, in the morning and at bedtime.

Athlete's foot, which is a fungus infection, can be treated with Desenex® or Tinactin® ointment and powders. **Eczema** can be treated with over-the-counter cortisone preparations. Many times, eczema of the feet can resemble tinea, a fungal disease of the skin, but eczema does not respond to anti-fungal treatment. If you suspect you have eczema, try cortisone; however, if the condition is very severe, try to track down its cause. A detergent used to wash the socks or a chemical used in the manufacture of your shoes, activated by sweat, may be the culprit.

If there is no improvement after a few weeks of treatment, seek medical help.

Muscle Cramps

In the *New England Journal of Medicine*, Dr. Harry Daniell described a technique for relieving cramps in the calf of the leg with an easy stretching motion.[1]

---

[1] H.W. Daniell, "Simple Care for Nocturnal Leg Cramps" (letter), *New England Journal of Medicine* 298, no. 19 (May 11, 1978): 1089–90.

Recurrent cramps in forty-five adults were controlled by this method within one week, and all victims remained cramp-free for more than a year with no further treatment.

The stretching exercise consists of leaning forward while facing a wall two to three feet away, using the hands and arms to regulate the forward tilt, and keeping heels in contact with the floor while leaning. This position creates a moderately intense pulling sensation in the calf muscle. The position is held for ten seconds twice, with a five-second rest between maneuvers, and then repeated three times daily until all leg cramps cease.

These exercises are best done after a vigorous hike or jog. They will also help if your leg cramps are caused by a potassium deficiency. Another possible cause is dehydration, especially in older individuals. It is easier to carry the fluids in your belly than on your back, so keep drinking during the hike. If the cramps occur while driving home, get out of the car and walk; if on a bus or train, walk up and down the aisle until you have relief.

Allergies
Allergies encountered outdoors are annoying but are not generally life-threatening. If cold weather or physical exertion causes chest congestion and wheez-

ing, medications can help.

Frequent bouts of sneezing or tearing may be due to pollen. Carry some antihistamines—they may give you a bit of relief. If your eyes tend to get very itchy, ask your medical facility for eye drops, so you can administer them directly in order to counter this allergic manifestation. The antihistamine eye preparations are safe but not always effective. Cortisone preparations are very effective but require medical supervision.

Seldane®, Hismanal®, and Claritin® are antihistamines used for allergic rhinitis (inflammation of the mucous membranes in the nose), but they require a prescription and not everyone can take them—ask your doctor. Seldane® is taken twice a day. Claritin® and Hismanal® are taken once a day. None of these drugs causes drowsiness, which is a problem with most other antihistamines.

Benadryl® does the same thing as Seldane®, but it is associated with drowsiness. However, it is less expensive, and if it is taken at bedtime, the drowsiness it induces can be an asset.

If you have food allergies, make certain that the gorp you are eating does not contain a food item that makes you break out. The same rule applies to the famous one-dish backpacking meals that contain everything except the kitchen sink.

If you are allergic to feathers, don't buy goose- or duck-down clothing or sleeping bags. Don't share a tent with another occupant using a goose-down bag.

People with bronchial asthma have usually had previous attacks and have learned to manage the problem. If you have asthma, consult your physician for advice and medications before embarking on a trip.

With the availability of cortisone, antihistamines, bronchodilators, and adrenaline, there is no reason allergies should prevent you from hiking.

(For information on allergic reactions to insect bites and stings, see pages 63ff.)

Colds

Colds can make you miserable, but they don't have to keep you off the trail. There are ways to deal with the discomfort so you can keep hiking.

You can carry a few four-milligram tablets of Chlortrimeton® (which can be purchased without a prescription) in your first-aid kit. Some preparations of Chlortrimeton® have an antihistamine plus a decongestant, such as Tavist-D® (OTC). Some recent studies have questioned the efficacy of Chlortrimeton®, while others have praised it. In two letters in the *Journal of the American Medical Association* (October 20, 1993), for example, one group argues that Chlortrimeton® is effective, while another group feels that studies citing its efficacy are flawed. The controversy continues.

Decongestant nose drops are effective. If you dislike nose drops and prefer an oral medication, try Sudafed®, but be sure to read the warning labels.

Megadoses of vitamin C are not effective as either a preventative or a cure for colds. Since a cold is a self-limited disease, do whatever your heart desires. You're going to get better no matter what!

Constipation

Whenever the topic of regularity comes up, the stress is usually on diarrhea or its treatment. But while climbing one summer in the Sawtooth Mountains, I realized that some members of the Iowa Mountaineers were having the opposite problem.

If you tend to be constipated on trips, carry some Senokot-S® tablets, which can be purchased over-the-counter. The usual dosage is two tablets twice a day, which you can increase to a maximum of four tablets twice a day if necessary. At proper dosage levels, Senokot-S® is virtually free of side effects.

A high-fiber diet can help you avoid constipation; eat bran, fresh fruits and vegetables, salads, and whole wheat and rye breads. Some people swear by figs, prunes, and fruit juices—especially prune and apple juice.

(For information on diarrhea, see page 95.)

Rucksack Palsy

In 1975, staff members of the Cleveland Clinic Foundation described a case of a 15-year-old boy who complained of left shoulder pain for two weeks.[1] Before the onset of the pain, he had been hiking and wore a rucksack with contents weighing about 45 pounds. He wore the pack for about six hours a day for seven days. During that time, he experienced some pain in his left arm and shoulder, but not enough to slow him down.

Examination revealed some wasting of the left deltoid and left biceps muscle, and damage of nerves in the brachial plexus, a group of nerves in the shoulder area. The damage required a graduated exercise program in order to be corrected. It took two months to achieve normal function and six months for the muscle bulk to return to normal.

Over the years, other similar incidents have been reported sporadically. A 1968 article in *Pediatrics* described the same type of condition experienced by several Boy Scouts. In 1969, J.R. Daube reported on 17 victims who suffered damage to the brachial plexus while wearing heavy packs.[2]

---

[1]*Pediatrics* 56, no. 5 (November 1975): 822–24.

[2]J.R. Daube, "Rucksack Paralysis," *Journal of the American Medical Association* 208, no. 13 (June 30, 1969): 2447–52.

With the increase in the use of backpacks and rucksacks, we can expect to see more widespread damage like that described above. It is estimated that nearly four million people are involved in hiking, climbing, and backpacking, and they all wear packs.

To prevent the problem, don't use your rucksack to do a backpack's job. The rucksack was not intended for extremely heavy weights. The backpack, if properly designed, puts the load on the back and hips while sparing the shoulders.

If you feel pain or a peculiar sensation when using a rucksack, do something about it immediately. Don't wait until you're really suffering. If possible, lighten the load. If you cannot, support the bottom of the pack to alleviate the pressure on the shoulders. Try adjusting the shoulder straps to give you more comfort. Put on your sweater or parka, weather permitting, to give your underarm area more padding.

Occasionally, hands become swollen while wearing a pack. The condition is benign, however. Raise your hands over your head, and open and close them repeatedly until the swelling subsides. It may look silly, but it's preferable to having swollen hands.

The problem can also occur with backpacks, but it happens less frequently. If it does, stop and readjust your straps and waist belt. Prevention is the best cure.

Toothaches
While not life-threatening, toothaches may make you
wish for death instead of the pain. Take an analgesic
such as aspirin; take two tablets every four hours until
you get help. Ice, if available, should be applied. If
you know you have a potential problem, get a prescription for a pain killer from your dentist before you
hit the trail. If all else fails, and the weather is warm
(or your hike is over and you're inside), turn to drink.
Swish some whiskey around the problem tooth (but be
aware that some of it is bound to be ingested). Repeat
this procedure several times. The pain should diminish.
If you are prone to toothaches, put some eugenol or
oil of cloves in your first-aid kit. They are also good for
relieving toothache pain, and help maintain some
degree of sobriety.

John C. Hall, M.D., who is active with the Appalachian Trail community in Georgia, suggests carrying
dental floss, which has many uses. For instance, you
can use it to splint one tooth against another in dental
injuries.

CHAPTER TWO
The Environment

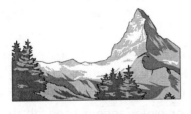 Broadly speaking, the environment is home to hikers everywhere. As wondrous and beautiful as it is, however, the environment is also home to some elements that are not always friendly to humans. If you want to hike, you should learn how to share the environment with other creatures, and how to adapt to the vicissitudes of the outdoors.

Cold Weather
Under proper conditions, winter activities can be enjoyable, but frozen feet and hands, as well as chills—brought about by heat loss—can detract from the joy. The four horsemen of heat loss are radiation,

conduction, convection, and vaporization.

Radiation is the emission or absorption of heat energy. The body radiates heat to nearby solid objects that have a cooler temperature. **Conduction** is the transfer of heat from the body by direct contact (with wet clothing, cold ground, metal, etc.). **Convection** is heat loss caused by contact with air or water that is colder than the body temperature (wind chill). **Vaporization** heat loss occurs when perspiration is converted to a gas (sweating).

Common Injuries from Cold

Injuries from cold temperatures can occur at any time of the year. You can meet winter conditions during the summer at high altitudes or experience a snowfall in New Hampshire's White Mountains or the Canadian Rockies in August.

Heat loss via wet clothing—as well as contact with cold ground, with rocks, or with metals, wind chill, and radiation—all increase the risk of cold injury, as do exhaustion, hunger, and alcohol consumption. Alcohol may curb shivering, the involuntary mechanism that produces heat, and it draws body heat away from the extremities. Drinking an alcoholic beverage when it is cold is like shooting yourself in the foot.

Avoid wearing cotton clothing in cold weather. It has a chilling effect when wet. Wool and polypropylene retain their ability to insulate even in wet conditions.

There are several types of injury from the cold, none of them pleasant and some worse than others. The most common ones are **hypothermia, frostbite**, and **frostnip**. **Chilblains** and **trench foot** are other injuries caused by the cold.

Hypothermia

Hypothermia can occur when you get wet either from outside your clothing because of rain, snow, wet foliage, and so forth, or from underneath your clothing through perspiration, improper apparel (see "Clothing for Cold Weather," page 39), overexhaustion, chilling, and consumption of improper foods and beverages. A high-carbohydrate diet is desirable, and preferable to a diet high in fat. If you have no choice, however, eat what is available. Consume as much fluid as possible—water, tea, soup, coffee, soda—but do not drink alcohol. Consuming as much fluid as possible *before* and *during* a hike is helpful in avoiding cold injuries and hypothermia.

> *Be aware of the condition, be prepared for the situation, and start doing something about it before it's too late.*

Hypothermia—The Silent Killer

Four of us were in the Adirondacks doing Mt. Dix on a rainy but not overly cold day in October. Rain and cold-weather gear made us uncomfortably hot and sweaty. After a few "shedding stops," we reached the summit and were greeted with cold, wet, gale-like winds.

In very short order, two of us started shivering; my feet became uncomfortably cold in my wet boots. I had problems working the toggle on my pack and getting my mittens. We all agreed that we'd better get off the summit before we froze to death.

We descended as fast as we could to a sheltered area, changed, and put on all the clothing we had in our packs. We ate chocolate and drank Wyler's and Tang. Life became more tolerable. Fortunately, we recognized the early stages of hypothermia, and avoided a tragedy.

Despite a lot of publicity about the dangers of hypothermia, hikers continue to be victims of this silent killer. An eerie presence fills the site of the former Montray Shelter on the Appalachian Trail in North Carolina, where a hiker died from hypothermia in 1986.

At a Royal Air Force Institute meeting some years ago, a story was told of sixteen men on a whaling vessel that capsized off the coast of Greenland in extremely cold Arctic waters. When rescued, all were able to climb the netting to board the rescue ship, partake of hot drinks, and get under blankets. But all sixteen died, due to "rewarming collapse"—a failure of the heart to function, which is associated with hypothermia.

Hypothermia victims, except in mild cases, should be hospitalized as soon as possible.

Carry as much extra clothing as you can, such as dry socks, mittens, and sweaters. The important thing is to be aware of the condition, be prepared for the situation, and start doing something about it before it's too late.

Hypothermia can be lethal, and it does not require below-freezing temperatures to develop. The danger is also present when the temperature is in the 50s and 60s. In fact, in the higher temperatures, hikers are more often lulled into a false sense of security; in very cold weather, hikers tend to dress adequately. When protected, you can tolerate environmental temperatures of –50 degrees, but a drop of seven degrees in your core, or inner, body temperature is dangerous in any weather.

Hypothermia occurs when the body loses more heat than it can produce and the core temperature begins to drop. If the drop in temperature is not halted, death can ensue in a few hours. Shivering is usually the first manifestation of hypothermia, and it stops when the core temperature falls below the range of 90–92° F. When shivering stops, the victim is in deep trouble.

Other signs of hypothermia include difficulty in using your hands, stumbling, losing articles of clothing, and behaving in a bizarre manner. This is followed by speech deficiency, blurred thinking, and amnesia. The shivering is eventually replaced by muscle rigidity, accompanied by stupor and drowsiness. When the core temperature falls below 78 degrees, cardiac and respiratory failure occur, and then death. The insidious aspect of hypothermia is the drowsiness and stupor, often leading to sleep.

Treating Hypothermia. The treatment for hypothermia, if you or your companions experience any of its symptoms, is to find the most sheltered spot available, boil water and drink hot liquids, and eat candy, gorp, and granola. If hot liquids are not available, drink what you have, but avoid all forms of alcohol. Alcohol is a vasodilator and causes greater heat loss.

If you have a tent, use it. It is a good idea to carry a tube tent for emergency bivouac. It is light and inexpensive, and can accommodate three people in a pinch. If there is snow on the ground and you can find a sheltered spot, dig a snow cave—it gives superb protection. Try to keep active to increase heat production.

If you have a sleeping bag, get out of all wet clothes and get into the bag. If at all possible, build a fire. Stay in the sleeping bag and near the fire until you feel your body temperature is normal. If you have a stove available, start heating your sweetened juices and drink them as hot as possible. However, *if you are inside a tent, make sure that you provide for a suffi-cient amount of ventilation*, no matter how bitterly cold it is outside. Without the proper ventilation, you will encounter the problem of **asphyxia**, which is caused by using a stove inside a closed area and burning up your available oxygen. Ensuring adequate ventilation also minimizes the condensation of mois-ture inside the tent and helps keep your equipment and clothing dry.

Frostnip and Frostbite
Frostnip, which can occur when you are exposed to temperatures around freezing (32 degrees F.), is a superficial injury that leaves firm, white areas, usually on the hands, feet, and parts of the face. It is treated by rapid warming with the hands, if they are not affected, or with a warm object, such as a stone that has been near the campfire, or a handwarmer. If the hands are affected, place them under your armpits or in your groin. Do not rub them with snow. Thaw the frozen parts gradually—stay away from hot fires. If your feet are involved, convince someone to allow you to warm them on his or her abdomen. If a sleeping bag is available, climb in.

In **frostbite**, which is more serious than frostnip and can occur when the temperature drops below freezing, the affected part of the skin is cold, white, hard, and completely numb. On rewarming, the area becomes blotchy, red, painful, and swollen. If it is a mild case, you may get off scot-free. If it is severe, gangrene is possible; gangrenous tissue feels cold and turns black in color. The first-aid treatment is the same as that for frostnip (see above), but it is even more important to get professional help immediately in the case of frostbite. Severe exposure is an absolute emergency. Until then, use a sleeping bag with someone else in it to provide external heat.

Chilblains and Trench Foot

Exposure around or above freezing can also cause chilblains and trench foot. **Chilblains** is a nonfreezing cold injury that does not cause damage but can be uncomfortable. The skin becomes red, itchy, warm, tender, and somewhat swollen. It can be treated by applying skin moisturizers; warm clothing prevents its occurrence. **Trench foot** is a cold injury to the feet caused by prolonged exposure to cold, wet weather. It was first observed among infantry soldiers who had spent a great deal of time in the trenches, which were wet and cold. When the body becomes cold, circulation to the feet is impaired because of vasoconstriction (the body's way of preserving heat); this brings about tissue damage. Tingling in the feet due to nerve damage is a prominent symptom of trench foot. The skin becomes red; this is followed by the appearance of blisters, bleeding under the skin, and swelling. The treatment is to elevate the feet in a warm environment. Severe cases require hospitalization.

Clothing for Cold Weather

At one time, wool and down (usually goose down) were the fabrics of choice for hiking clothes. Goose-down garments are very efficient in preventing heat loss; they are highly compressible and they weigh very little. A good goose-down parka and sleeping bag are expensive, but they are well worth the money as long as they are kept dry. If down gets wet, however, it is worthless. Therefore, if you are doing any kind of *active* hiking in cold weather, you should probably avoid goose down, as it is bound to get wet when you perspire. In addition, rain and snow make for a dangerous environment if your gear is not protected.

In recent years, there has been a proliferation of synthetics such as polypropylene, Capilene®, and others, which broaden your selection. The synthetics are less expensive than wool and down, and not itchy like wool. They also wick the moisture away from the body, which is important in cold weather especially, because staying dry is crucial to prevent heat loss.

Dressing in Cold Weather

Certain axioms of dressing for cold weather can make the difference as to whether you enjoy winter hiking or resign yourself to hiking in warm weather exclusively. They can also prevent serious injury.

—*Do* layer your clothing: Dressing in multiple layers of thin clothing is more efficient than wearing one bulky garment, because it allows you to peel off successive layers as you become warm, and put them back on one by one as you become cold.

—*Do* use wind pants and a shirt made from wool or one of the newer synthetic materials; they block cold air and reduce heat loss due to convection.

—*Do* wear a button-down shirt, which can be unbuttoned if you become overheated.

—*Do* wear clothes made of fabrics that wick away moisture, such as polypropylene, Capilene®, or silk.

—*Don't* wear turtlenecks if you are physically active, because they trap heat.

—*Don't* wear cotton clothing in cold weather, because it does not retain warmth and, once wet, it tends to stay wet. Denim, in particular, is heavy, retains moisture, and seems to stay wet forever. Don't even wear cotton underwear—choose wool, silk, or a synthetic, such as polypropylene or Capilene®, instead.

—*Don't* wear sneakers in cold weather.

—*Don't* overdress: perspiring can lead to hypothermia.

Tips for Fending Off the Cold

Dr. Murray Hamlet, who gave a lecture tour in Nepal, discussed some unusual hints for fending off the cold never mentioned in the typical mountaineering literature:

— Men should shave at night rather than in the morning, to give the facial oils, which fight dry skin, a chance to return by morning. Shaving peels the outer layer of skin, and in dry, cold air, it results in dry, raw skin. Or, use a hand cream on the face. Growing a beard solves the whole problem.

— To prevent or heal chapped hands, use a cream with a fish-oil base, such as Desitin® or A&D Cream®, and at night, sleep with thin cotton gloves on your hands.

— Avoid jewelry, because metal conducts cold. Earrings are the greatest problem, and pierced earrings, particularly, bring cold to the ears. Metal eyeglass frames conduct cold as well, and they separate the ear from the head. Dr. Hamlet says people who wear glasses are more prone to frostbite of the ears than those who do not.

— Thick soles and anything that will keep your feet off the cold ground will help keep your feet warm.

— Suspenders are better than tight belts, which may hamper the movement of warm air.

— A thimbleful of olive oil in the last rinse when washing woolens keeps them from scratching.

Although the synthetics are not as lightweight or compressible as goose down, they retain their insulating capability when wet.

If you are allergic to wool and/or feathers, the synthetics are the way to go. If you can't tolerate synthetics either, restrict the locale of your winter activities to the Virgin Islands.

Remember to keep your clothing dry so the insulating qualities are retained. If you do become wet, move as rapidly as possible to create more body heat, and change into dry clothes as soon as possible.

Legs and Feet

Knickers have some advantage over trousers: You can roll down your stockings if you are overheated, and you can open the bottom fasteners and roll up the legs, if necessary. Woolen trousers, or Polarguard® tights or pants, are also good in cold weather. They dry out quickly and retain their insulating properties even when wet.

If cold feet are a problem, wear insulated boots such as Sorels® or L.L. Bean® boots with felt or Thinsulate® liners. Plastic boots are warm, but they don't accommodate the foot as well as leather and, of course, they don't breathe. "Mickey Mouse" boots, which were used during the Korean War, create a vapor barrier that insulates feet against the cold.[1] Some of the vapor barrier boots can have air pumped into them to increase the insulation. Neoprene® socks, which also help to retain heat, are expensive but they render a service well worth their cost.

You can make a vapor barrier inside your own boots if they are roomy enough. Wear a light pair of woolen or synthetic socks with a plastic bag over them, and cover the bag with one or two pairs of moderately heavy wool or synthetic socks. Vapor barrier lock socks are available in mountaineering stores. I have not used them, but I understand that they may irritate the foot, since they do not fit smoothly, and moisture can macerate (weaken) the skin. They are useful in an emergency when feet get wet. There are neoprene attachments that you can put over your toes if they tend to be cold.

Not all boots accommodate crampons. If you plan on using crampons, make sure that the boot is rigid enough for them before you make your purchase.

Gaiters are another modality for conserving heat. They not only insulate, but aid in keeping the feet dry.

---

[1] I have been unable to account for the origin of the name "Mickey Mouse" boots. David R. Smith, an archivist at the Walt Disney Company, was unfamiliar with the term, but he speculated that it could be a reference to the cartoon character's unusually oversized shoes.

As an added bonus, they help keep your socks clean. Insulated inner soles, if they can accommodate your foot, also help.

Face and Hands
If cold hands are a problem, mittens are warmer than gloves. If you want the best of both worlds, wear thin silk, polypropylene, or light woolen gloves with insulated down or pile mittens over them, so you have some protection if you have to use your fingers. Insulating the trunk makes heat loss from the hands more tolerable, too. (Years ago I purchased a pair of Eddie Bauer's expedition mittens. These were down-filled and insulated. On the back of the mitten, there is a patch of goat fur, which you can use to wipe a runny nose. Blowing your nose in subzero weather becomes a challenge. Handkerchiefs become stiff as a board in no time flat.)

A wool, polypropylene, or synthetic pile face mask comes in handy on a bitter, blustery day. A balaclava can be pulled down to give some protection to the face.

Using Your Head to Conserve Heat
Freezing various and sundry parts of your anatomy does not lend itself to happiness and can be downright dangerous. For heat conservation, use your head.

Going through life with a cool head is great, but don't overdo it on a cold, wintery day. *Wear a hat.* A balaclava, mentioned above, is ideal for this situation. The head is 5 percent of the body surface, but you can lose 40 percent of your body heat through your head, including the ears. Ear muffs are of great help, but if it is cold enough for ear muffs, you're better off with a hat. There is an old adage: "If your feet are cold, wear a hat."

There is an old adage: "If your feet are cold, wear a hat."

The amount of heat conservation needed to stay warm varies from one individual to another. Some people can tolerate cold much better than others because of genes, sex, age, alcohol use, circulation, and weight. So, customize when you winterize!

Hot Weather

If you have a streak of masochism in your makeup, don't be concerned about leaving the problems of cold weather behind you: hot weather has its own special offerings to make you miserable. I don't know what George Gershwin had in mind when he wrote, "Summer time and the living is easy."

Problems from Too Much Heat

Sunstroke, also known as **heat stroke**, is the most serious problem of the lot. The symptoms are similar to heat prostration but the pulse rate can be over 160, whereas in heat prostration it is usually below 100. (A normal pulse range is 60–90.) The body temperature rises to over 105 degrees Fahrenheit. Convulsions and vomiting may follow. Cool the victim off the best you can and get to a hospital. Do not allow the temperature to go below 101 degrees F., so the patient does not go from hyperthermia to hypothermia.[1]

Heat prostration, also called **heat exhaustion**, occurs from exposure to excessive heat, with prostration and circulatory collapse. It is manifested by listlessness, apprehension, and, in severe cases, unconsciousness. The skin becomes ashen, cold, and wet, with profuse perspiration. Symptoms consist of

---

[1]Dr. Charles S. Houston, who wrote the section on sunstrokes in the *Merck Manual* (16th edition, 1992), notes that, to prevent hyperthermia from turning into hypothermia, one should stop reducing the victim's temperature when it reaches 101 degrees, since the temperature-regulating mechanism is extremely labile in sunstroke victims (p. 2510). William Forgey's *Wilderness Manual* notes that U.S. Steel Mill treated the victims of heat stroke (sunstroke) by immersing them in ice water until their temperature dropped to 102 degrees, and then carefully monitored the temperature, because it could either keep falling or start rising again.

weakness, dizziness, headache, and blurred vision. If the victim can be given oral hydration, this is the route to go. If not possible, then the patient should be taken to a hospital for intravenous therapy. To prevent the problem, keep as cool as possible and take an adequate amount of salt. Assuming that you do not have a problem with high blood pressure, supplement your salt intake with salted nuts and pretzels, and by adding salt to your sandwich.

Heat cramps are most common during the summer. Heat cramps in the legs are caused by an accumulation of lactic acid in the muscles and a great deal of perspiration, with its accompanying salt loss. The cramps appear suddenly, usually after several hours of strenuous hiking. The treatment is to rest and allow the blood to carry away the lactic acid. Deep breathing and stretching the cramped muscles, along with salt tablets, give relief. If you are perspiring excessively, take salt tablets as a preventive. If the ordinary salt tablets upset your stomach, get the enteric-coated salt tablets. As mentioned above, you can also supplement your salt intake with salted nuts and pretzels, and by adding salt to your sandwich. (If you have high blood pressure, don't go overboard on the salt without consulting your physician.)

Other, more minor problems are rashes, which are not life-threatening but can be very annoying. **Miliaria**, better known as heat rash, is brought about by the obstruction of the sweat glands. It is caused by excessive perspiration in a hot environment. Obese hikers are the most susceptible to this type of rash. If large numbers of sweat glands become obstructed, the regulation of body heat may be impaired. The problem disappears if sweating stops, so if you develop a heat rash, stop exerting yourself and find a cool environment with low-calorie food.

Intertrigo is a chafing caused by moisture, warmth, and two skin surfaces rubbing together, resulting in burning and irritation. Obesity and hot weather are important predisposing factors. To resolve the problem, keep cool, try to lose weight, and use a cortisone ointment or any soothing ointment if cortisone is not available.

If all else fails, find a nice, cool, air-conditioned bar; replenish your fluids with beer; and compensate for your salt depletion with potato chips, salted peanuts, and pretzels.

Sunburn
The most common type of burn experienced by hikers, skiers, swimmers, and even glacier strollers is sunburn. Although generally associated with hot weather, sunburn can occur at any time of the year. The concept of "preventive tanning" by using an ultraviolet

sun lamp or "tanning booth" before sun exposure is invalid. It gives zero protection, and it results in permanent damage to the skin.

The increased use of sunscreening agents has reduced the incidence and severity of sunburn, but it is still common. In fact, the use of sunscreens can give us a false sense of security, because they do not provide complete protection against sunburn. (Only a true sun *block*—such as zinc oxide ointment or pants and a long-sleeved shirt—can provide total protection.)

Any sunscreen's effect varies depending on its sun protection factor, or SPF. The higher the SPF, the more chemicals in the sunscreen, and the more protection. An SPF of 8 allows you to stay in the sun eight times longer than you could normally tolerate. So if you usually burn after ten minutes of exposure, a sunscreen with an SPF of 8 protects you for eighty minutes.

If you are out in the sun for a long time, use a sunscreen religiously. A sunscreen with an SPF of 15 or higher will offer the best protection. (SPFs above 25, however, are probably meaningless in terms of offering extra protection; it's more likely they're a marketing ploy of the sunscreen manufacturers.) If you are very fair-skinned and/or burn easily, use a sunscreen with a high SPF, or a sun block. Reapply often, especially after swimming, towel drying, and sweating. Use zinc oxide to further protect the nose and lips.

You can get a sunburn while in the water, even on cloudy days. Beware of cool breezes under a strong sun; the breeze reduces the discomfort of burning, so you may not realize you're getting burned. Remember that ultraviolet rays bounce off sand, snow, glaciers, and cement, thus getting you from above and below. Also, the higher the altitude, the greater the exposure.

Treatment of Sunburn

The treatment for and prevention of extensive sunburn (and other types of burns, as well) includes cool baths, wet compresses, or, if available, ice packs. If you wear a ring, remove it, because tissues tend to get swollen and rings become very tight, and at times impossible to remove. The same holds true for bracelets.

Take adequate fluids to replace water loss, and replenish electrolyte loss by drinking Gatorade®. You can make your own brand with a solution of one-half level teaspoon of salt, 2 ounces of white Karo® syrup (clear), 8 ounces of orange juice, and 22 ounces of water. If possible, include fresh or dehydrated bananas in your diet; they help maintain the body's chemical balance.

Two aspirin every four hours may alleviate some of the pain caused by sunburn, and if there is an antihistamine around, take it, unless you have to drive. Topical cortisone ointments are no more effective than cold tap-water compresses. Avoid the use of anesthetic lotions and ointments that can sensitize the skin. If the burn is extensive enough to cause fever and chills, get professional help.

The main thrust of the treatment for and prevention of sunburn is to avoid any unnecessary exposure to the sun. This can best be done at the nearest bar and grill, which offers a cool, dark environment, ice-cold fluids to maintain a fluid balance, and pretzels to provide salt.

Skin Cancer

Several years ago, I received a letter from an old-time hiker asking me to write something about the dangers of sun exposure. He had developed a basal-cell cancer of an ear lobe. He was quite shocked, he said, since he lived right, exercised, watched his cholesterol, and took vitamins. It never occurred to him that he could get cancer from exposure to the sun.

The long-term effects of overexposure to the sun are more devastating than sunburn and harder to treat. The problem is that exposure results in radiation poisoning to the skin, which causes cell alterations and leads to cancer. As a preventive measure, the use of sunscreens should start in childhood, but it is never too late to start.

Water

> *"Water, water, everywhere,*
> *Nor any drop to drink."*
> —Samuel Taylor Coleridge,
> THE RIME OF THE ANCIENT MARINER

We all lead sane, orderly, civilized lives of some sort or other until we hit the trail. Then something happens to us. In the city, we would never dream of sharing our glass of water at a dinner party or in a restaurant, but on a hike or backpack, sharing a canteen is a common practice. If someone has not brought a beverage, it is embarrassing not to be a kind soul, a good sport, a decent human being— so we share our beverage along with our bacteria and our viruses.

Don't depend on other hikers to fulfill your thirst requirements.

Don't depend on other hikers to fulfill your thirst requirements. Don't expose yourself, and don't put anyone else in the position of feeling compelled to share. Shakespeare must have had this situation in mind when he said, "Neither a borrower nor a lender be." If you insist on mouth-to-mouth transmission of disease, do it by kissing. From personal experience, it is a much more pleasant mode of acquiring an illness. If you are a compulsive scrounger, at least bring your own cup. Have the same standards of good manners on the trail as you would have at home.

Day trips generally do not require communal cooking. We usually bring food from home for the lunch stop. However, on backpack trips and expeditions, group cooking is the usual modus operandi for food preparation, and the longer the trip, the greater the incidence of diarrhea and possibly vomiting. Here we run into the hand transmission of disease. The gourmet chef of the moment uses his finger to test the warmth of his delicacy, or his finger becomes the substitute for a tasting spoon. At best, the washing facilities on extended trips leave much to be desired. There are times when even those of us who want to wash have no facilities. Once you are made the chef for the occasion, try to remember the sign in the restaurant reminding employees to wash their hands after using the facilities. Cooking over a Svea®, an Optimus®, or an open fire does not impart immunity. If you think it does, I suggest you pack an adequate supply of toilet tissue.

Aqua Pura Revisited

Perhaps a better heading for this section would be "Don't Eat Yellow Snow or Drink It When It Melts." I continually receive requests for guidance in procuring safe water. I have a strong feeling that it is hard to accept the fact that the cool, bubbling, clear water flowing over the rocks in Torne Brook or Stony Brook or any other brook may be detrimental to your health. I have done some sampling in various popular areas, however (Baby Brook on Schunemunk Mountain in New York, the Weis Ecology Center in New Jersey, the New Jersey Wyanokies, and Stony Brook in New York's Harriman-Bear Mountain State Park), and I have found *Escherichia coli (E. coli)* bacteria, which indicate a possibility of fecal contamination.

I recall an outbreak of diarrhea that was experienced in a popular ski resort one winter. The water supply, fed by underground springs, was contaminated with harmful bacteria. The source of the contamination remained a mystery until someone decided to dump a dye in the johns that were located at the top of the various ski lifts surrounding the village. Lo and behold, the dye appeared in the water supply. The source was one latrine, which drained into a spring. The removal of this latrine solved the problem.

The fact is, with the tremendous outdoor population explosion that has taken place in the past twenty years, the odds are that most streams and lakes are contaminated. Work on the assumption that there is no such thing as "pure" water, and that all water requires treatment. The old adage about an ounce of prevention and a pound of cure applies to this situation. Why run the risk?

Of all the water organisms, *Giardia lamblia* is the most difficult to eliminate. It thrives in cold water, and complete elimination of the organism is essential. It is estimated that up to 20 percent of the population are carriers of this cyst. *Giardia* has been found in numerous animals, including beavers, deer, cats, dogs, cattle, and squirrels. Giardiasis has been called "beaver fever."

The best advice for day hikers is that they should bring their own drinks. For overnight backpackers, boiling the water is the safest procedure, but if that is not practical, the chemical disinfection methods described below can be used.

By the way, you don't have to be an outdoors person to get giardiasis: world travelers are eligible, too. St. Petersburg (Leningrad), Costa Del Sol, and Banff all have had *Giardia* in their water at some time or other.

Water Purification
There are several ways of handling the water situation. The options are boiling, chemical purification, or using a portable water purifier.

Boiling

Boiling water is safe and practical. One minute of boiling destroys *Giardia* cysts and bacteria, and 10 minutes will kill other organisms involved in water-borne disease. At high altitudes, boil water for 10 minutes. However, if there are many hikers in the party, boiling gallons of water becomes time-consuming, not to mention fuel-consuming, if gasoline, kerosene, or alcohol are the fuels. If snow is the only source of water at high altitudes, melt it and treat it chemically. At high altitudes, fuel is too precious a commodity to use for prolonged boiling of water.

Chemical Disinfection

Chemical disinfection, which has been used for years, is still a practical and convenient approach. The Environmental Protection Agency (EPA) recommends the chemical disinfection methods shown in Table 2.1.

Even though the EPA does not recommend the saturated iodine crystals method, I am not sure it should be discarded. Their objection is that it does not destroy *Giardia* in cold water. The original article[1] advocating its use recommended that the temperature

---

[1]F.H. Kahn and B.R. Visscher, "Water Disinfection in the Wilderness: A Simple, Effective Method of Iodination," *Western Journal of Medicine* 122 (May 1975): 450–53.

of the water be 77 degrees or more. However, other studies have shown that the saturated iodine crystals do destroy *Giardia* at 68 degrees, so if you are treating cold water, do it at night and take your canteen or water bottle into your sleeping bag. During the day, carry it in a pocket or under your jacket until it warms up, or place it near your fire or in the sun.

Table 2.1
The EPA's Recommended Methods for the Chemical Disinfection of Water

Disinfectant	Quantity per quart	Waiting time before drinking
Chlorine tablet	5 tablets	30 minutes[a]
Household bleach	4 drops	30 minutes
Iodine tablets	2 tablets	20 minutes[a]
2% tincture of iodine	10 drops	20 minutes
Saturated iodine crystals	Not recommended	—

[a]For tablets, the waiting time begins after the tablets dissolve.
Source: Environmental Protection Agency

To use the **iodine crystals**, place eight grams of the crystals in a one-ounce clear glass bottle with a plastic cap. If you can get your pharmacist to give you a calibrated bottle, so much the better. Fill the bottle with water and shake vigorously for 30 seconds. Allow the crystals to settle, then decant 12.5 cc (five capfuls or a little less than half of the solution). Add this to a quart or liter of water to be treated, and allow to stand overnight if possible. If the water is above 68 degrees F., it can be used after 30 minutes. This method is inexpensive, the crystals do not deteriorate, and the solution provides at least a thousand applications. (See also the recommendations of the New Mexico Health and Environmental Department, below.)

Chlorine tablets, by contrast, which are sold as Halazone®, are not stable, have a short shelf life (five months), and lose their effectiveness when exposed to air or heat. (However, they can be used successfully, as described in the recommendations issued by the New Mexico Health and Environmental Department, below.) **Iodine tablets**, which are sold under various names—Globaline®, Potable Aqua®, Coughlan's EDWGT® (Emergency Drinking Water Germicidal Tablet)—lose 20 percent of their effectiveness when exposed to the air for four days. If you use iodine or chlorine tablets, make certain you take a fresh bottle on each trip and hope your supplier has a large turnover so the supplies are fresh.

The New Mexico Health and Environmental Department (NMHED) has issued one of the most comprehensive schemes I have seen for purifying water (including boiling, chlorination, and iodination). They recommend straining visibly dirty or cloudy water through a cloth to filter out debris or organic matter, before starting any disinfection process. Their guidelines for chemical disinfection differ somewhat from the EPA recommendations in that they are more specific and, in addition to describing the use of chlorine, iodine tablets, and tincture of iodine, they also recommend the use of iodine crystals.

To chlorinate, the NMHED recommends using either Halazone® tablets or common bleach. If Halazone® is used, start with an unopened bottle for each trip. Halazone® must be protected from the heat and from exposure to the air or it will become ineffective. Follow the directions on the label for use. If you use bleach, begin by reading the label to determine its percentage of chlorine. (Liquid chlorine laundry bleach usually has 4 to 6 percent available chlorine.) Then use as instructed in Table 2.2.

Mix thoroughly by stirring or shaking the water in the container, and let stand for 30 minutes. A slight chlorine odor should be detectable in the water; if it is not, repeat the dosage and let stand for an additional fifteen minutes before using. The water should then be safe to drink.

Table 2.2
Purifying Water with the Chlorination Method

Available chlorine	Drops[a] to add per quart or liter	
	Add to clear water	Add to cold or cloudy water[b]
1%	10	20
4–6%	2	4
7–10%	1	2
Unknown	10	20

[a]One drop = 0.05 ml.
[b]Very turbid or very cold water may require prolonged contact time; let stand for several hours or overnight.
Source: State of New Mexico, Health and Environmental Dep't.

The NMHED's recommendations for iodinating water include the use of Globaline® tablets, tincture of iodine, or iodine crystals. If Globaline® is used, begin with an unopened bottle on each trip. Globaline® must be protected from heat and from exposure to the air, or it will become ineffective. Follow directions for use on the Globaline® label.

Another method is to add five drops (one drop = 0.05 ml) of 2 percent tincture of iodine to each quart or liter of clear water, or 10 drops to each quart or liter of cold or cloudy water. (Very turbid or very cold water may require prolonged contact time; let stand for several hours or overnight.) Mix thoroughly by stirring or shaking the water in its container and let stand for 30 minutes.

Iodine crystals can be ordered from your pharmacy if they don't keep them in stock. The Kahn-Visscher (KV) method, recommended by the NMHED, is useful, but it requires some advance preparation. Begin by placing four to eight grams (about a quarter-ounce) of USP grade resublimed iodine in a one-ounce clear glass bottle with a leakproof cap. To purify water:

1 Fill the one-ounce bottle with water and shake it strongly for one minute.

2 Hold the bottle upright until the heavy iodine crystals settle to the bottom. The liquid is now a saturated iodine solution.

3 Determine the proper volume of the saturated iodine solution that must be added to each liter or quart of water (see Table 2.3).

4 Determine the amount of time you should wait between adding the saturated iodine solution and drinking the water; this depends both on the water's visible cleanliness and its temperature. Longer contact times help to ensure better disinfection; several hours or overnight are the most effective. If the water was heavily contaminated or is very cold, wait at least one hour. If you are

purifying relatively clean water that isn't very cold, you can drink it 30 minutes after adding the saturated iodine solution.

Table 2.3
Purifying Water with Iodine Crystals

Water temperature	Volume of saturated iodine to add per quart	Capfuls[a] of solution to add per quart
3° C. (37° F.)	20 cc	8–10
20° C. (68° F.)	13 cc	5–6
25° C. (77° F.)	12.5 cc	5
40° C. (104° F.)	10 cc	4

[a]A single capful from the one-ounce bottle will contain about 2.5 cc, so the cap can be used as a handy measuring device.
Source: State of New Mexico, Health and Environmental Department.

Water Filters

A third method of purification is a portable water filter, classified as a water purifier. Backpackers and people going on expeditions use water filters more frequently than do day hikers. My experience with portable water filters is limited, but they have faults. Some are ineffective, some are bulky, and many are expensive and time-consuming. Whatever water filter you choose, make certain that it removes *Giardia*, and keep in mind that in subfreezing temperatures water filters are useless.

Insect Bites and Stings

A batch of friendly, outgoing, gregarious insects as companions on a hike can be disconcerting, and on a backpack trip they can be an utter disaster. For those who are allergic to insect bites and stings, they can even be life-threatening.

There is no set figure on the incidence of insect-sting sensitivity; discrepancies exist depending upon geographic area, age of the subject, and life style.[1] The prime concern is the sting of the *Hymenoptera* order, which includes hornets, bees, yellow jackets, wasps, and ants. Theirs are the stings responsible for the most serious problems. However, on most hikes, when an

------

[1]"The frequency of insect sting allergy in a given population varies depending on . . . age group . . . and type of criteria used. . . . In a pediatric population with a mean age of 13 years, . . . the frequency is 0.8% using history as the only criteria. With this same criteria in an adult population, . . . the frequency [was] 3.3%. The difference is probably due to the prolonged exposure rate to insect stings in adults." G.A. Settipane and George K. Boyd, "Natural History of Insect Sting Allergy: The Rhode Island Experience," *Allergy Proceedings* (March–April 1989): 109.

insect is sighted, it is usually referred to as a bee. As an apiculturist, I take exception to this term: the stinging insects are usually not honey bees.

An insect sting can cause an immediate reaction, with symptoms ranging from mild swelling at the sting site, pain, and hives, to a tightness of the throat and chest (causing labored breathing), abdominal pain, nausea, vomiting, dizziness, difficulty in swallowing, hoarseness, thickened speech, and confusion. On rare occasions, these symptoms can be followed by shock associated with cyanosis (blueness of the skin), incontinence, and unconsciousness. Hikers with a known hypersensitivity to insect stings should not be on the trail without a personal first-aid kit for administering adrenaline (epinephrine), which includes a preloaded syringe of adrenaline, a tourniquet, and antihistamines. When the reactions create hives, wheezing, and a tightness of the chest and throat, the situation may be life-threatening. In such a case, an adrenaline injection should be administered, if possible, along with an antihistamine, and plans should be made to evacuate immediately and seek the nearest

> *Hikers with a known hypersensitivity to insect stings should not be on the trail without adrenaline.*

medical help. Adrenaline should be used with great caution as it is potentially dangerous if you have a heart condition.

If adrenaline is not available, and the sting is on an extremity, wrap a surgical bandage around and above the sting site. Do not make it too tight or it will cut off circulation. When you can, seek medical help.

The incidence of deaths from a stinging insect is very small. In all my years of hiking, I have never had an occasion to give an adrenaline injection.

Stings without generalized symptoms are not an indication for adrenaline. Local reactions are no cause for alarm. If you know you tend to be sensitive, carry an antihistamine, such as Benadryl® or Chlortrimeton®, which can be purchased over-the-counter; it may help counteract mild symptoms. If you develop hives and generalized itching after a sting, take an antihistamine and get to a medical facility as soon as possible. These symptoms are not life-threatening, but it is still advisable to seek medical guidance, even if the symptoms disappear, because the next sting has the potential of being lethal.

Tick-Borne Diseases

We have become so involved with Lyme disease of late that we tend to overlook the other diseases that are tick-borne. Just because a tick is not a Lyme-disease–carrying tick does not mean that you will get off scot-free. Even the ticks associated with the transmission of Lyme disease can transmit other diseases. The reassuring thought is that most of them are relatively rare.

Someone once described **Lyme disease** as a ticking time bomb, and it is an appropriate description. Until 1975, the only tick-borne disease of any note was Rocky Mountain Spotted Fever, and its incidence was relatively low in the northeastern United States. In fact, many people assumed it could be acquired only in the Rocky Mountains, since they knew of no one who had ever acquired it. Then Lyme disease was discovered in Lyme, Connecticut, after two mothers from that area became concerned when their children developed juvenile rheumatoid arthritis. In addition to their children, a whole cluster of similar cases was reported. The mothers could not accept the concept of an epidemic of juvenile rheumatoid arthritis, and insisted on an investigative study.

Lyme disease can be serious— but if treated early, the response is excellent.

The Yale Medical School was given the job, and their infectious disease people eventually determined that the infectious agent, a spirochete, *Borrelia burg-*

dorferi, was transmitted by the *Ixodes dammini* tick. We now know that other *Ixodes* ticks and the *Amblyomma Americanum* (Lone Star tick) can also be vectors. It was assumed that Lyme was a new disease, but it turned out that it had been described previously under different names; in the early 1900s it was called *erythema migrans* or *erythema chronicum migrans* (ECM), and in 1940 it was known as Bannwarth's disease. In time, it was learned that Lyme disease has been reported not only in Lyme, Connecticut, but in all the continents in the world except Antarctica. The incidence is greatest between May and November.

Many people contracting Lyme disease are not aware that they have been bitten by a tick. The first sign of the disease is a red pimple at the site of the tick bite. This is followed by an enlargement of the area of redness, and, generally, a raised border, usually within a week—but it can take as little as three days or as long as a month. The rash can range in size from one inch to twenty inches, and it creates a burning sensation. The rash usually fades within three to four weeks (with a range of one day to fourteen months).

Some victims do not get the rash at all, and in others the only symptom is the rash.[1] Some victims

---

[1] Allen C. Steere, who discovered Lyme disease, estimates that 20–40 percent of those infected do not develop a rash.

have a rash but don't see it, if it is on the back, behind the ears, behind the knees, or in the scalp. For others, any of the following symptoms can occur: fever, stiff neck, backache, muscle aches, sore throat, headache, nausea, and vomiting. Later, the acute phase complications can set in. These are cardiac abnormalities, joint pains associated with arthritis, and neurological diseases, including Bell's Palsy, or facial paralysis.

The recommended treatment is usually penicillin V, doxycycline, amoxicillin, or tetracycline for ten to thirty days. The Centers for Disease Control and Prevention stresses that early treatment can prevent or at least minimize the subsequent joint, neurological, and cardiac problems. So, if you've gotten a peculiar rash without being aware of having been bitten, see a doctor and explain that you think you may have Lyme disease. Don't wait for complications to set in.

Rocky Mountain spotted fever is also tick-borne; usually it is associated with the American dog tick (*Dermacentor variabilis*). However, it can also be transmitted by the Lone Star tick (which can also transmit Lyme disease). The infectious agent is *Rickettsia rickettsii*. The disease is widespread in both North and South America. The incidence is highest in July and August (the months most people go on vacation), and the number of reported cases has gone up dramatically since it was first identified. A likely cause for the increase, in addition to improved public and medical awareness, is the tremendous number of people taking to the woods and mountains in recent years for hiking, climbing, camping, and canoeing.

The rash differs from Lyme disease in that it consists of red spots under the skin, which appear two or three days after the fever starts. The ticks carrying the *Rickettsia* are active in the fall and winter as well as in the warm seasons. If you are bitten by a tick or experience a bug bite, and in a few days you develop a headache, loss of appetite, muscle aches, and joint pains, you may have contracted the spotted fever. These symptoms are followed by a rash that usually starts on the feet and ankles and spreads rapidly to the wrists and hands. It is accompanied by puffy eyes. See your doctor about the bite. Rocky Mountain spotted fever's status as an exotic entity in the Northeast will increase the doctor's index of suspicion.

Babesiosis is usually found in coastal areas, including Fire Island, Martha's Vineyard, and Shelter Island. The incidence is relatively low. It is caused by *Babesia microti*, which is a protozoa, and it resembles malaria in that it is manifested by a high fever, chills, and evidence of the parasite in the red blood cells. It is transmitted to humans through the bite of the nymphal *Ixodes dammini* tick, which is the same tick that is a vector for Lyme disease. I don't recall ever seeing any case studies that described a victim with Babesiosis *and* Lyme disease, but the possibility exists. Mild and asymptomatic Babesiosis infections do not require treatment. Quinine plus Clindamycin (Cleocin®) has been used in more serious infections. Babesiosis is most severe in people over 40 or those without a spleen. It is rarely fatal.

Ehrlichiosis is similar to Rocky Mountain spotted fever, with symptoms of chills, muscle pain, headache, joint pains, nausea, vomiting, loss of appetite, and weight loss. The rash that this disease causes is less prominent than the one seen in Rocky Mountain Spotted Fever. It starts about seven days after the onset of the illness, and it lasts one to two weeks. The causative agent is *Ehrlichia canis*, which is transmitted by ticks. It occurs May through July and is treated with tetracycline or chloramphenicol. It is usually found in the southern United States and on the east coast.

Borrelia (relapsing fever) shares two features with Lyme disease—both are caused by spirochetes and both are tick-borne. It has one advantage over Lyme disease: if you're lucky enough not to be bitten by an infected tick, you can still acquire it if you are bitten by an infected louse. The symptoms are headache, muscle pains, chills, high fever, joint pains, and a fleeting rash on the trunk. The disease lasts three to six days initially, is followed by a fever-free period for about a week, and then is followed by a relapse. The relapses are less severe than the first occurrence, and the fever-free period gets longer and longer; this cycle repeats itself until the disease disappears.

Borrelia is not easy to acquire. The ticks feed very briefly (about ten minutes, usually at night), so most victims are not aware of a tick bite. It is limited to the Rocky Mountain area and altitudes of 1,500–8,000 feet. It is certainly a very picky disease. Treatment consists of administering either tetracycline or chloramphenicol, to reduce the number of relapses.

Tularemia is caused by *Francisella tularemia*, which can be acquired from wild mammals, domestic animals, water, ticks, mosquitoes, and deerflies. The major carriers include the Lone Star tick, the dog tick, and rabbits. The incubation period for most cases is three to five days after exposure. The portal of entry is marked by a painful pimple, which eventually ulcerates. Victims can also develop painful, enlarged lymph glands and severe conjunctivitis. The treatment is gentamicin, chloramphenicol, or streptomycin. In addition to all the other precautions, don't handle any dead animals if you want to avoid this disease.

Colorado tick fever is caused by *Orbivirus*, and it entails two episodes of fever. It is found in the Rocky Mountain area and it is spread by the wood tick, *Dermacentor andersoni*. Three to five days after being bitten, the victim experiences fever, headache, chills, and muscle pains, with occasional abdominal pain, nausea, and vomiting. There may be a two- or three-day period without fever, and then fever recurs. Treatment involves acetaminophen or aspirin for fever, intravenous fluids for dehydration, vaseline for dry lips, and an ice bag to the forehead for headache. The illness lasts for about three weeks and then disappears.

Some ticks, after being attached to a person for several days, introduce a toxin that can induce **tick paralysis**, and that has a 10 percent mortality rate. Ascending paralysis develops four to seven days after tick attachment. Recovery takes place rapidly after the tick is removed. (See below, "Prevention and Tick Removal," for an explanation of how to properly remove a tick.)

Encephalitis is caused by *Flavivirus* and is transmitted by the *Ixodes* tick. It brings about an inflammation of the brain. The symptoms of encephalitis include severe headache, delirium, coma, seizures, nausea, vomiting, and death. Fortunately, it is rare. There is no one treatment for encephalitis; treatment depends upon where and when it occurs.

Prevention and Tick Removal

The usual advice for avoiding tick bites has been to wear long-sleeved shirts and pants, and to tuck the pant legs into the socks. Aside from the fact that such measures are not very realistic in 90-degree weather, some hikers now believe that, since ticks gravitate toward warm, moist, dark places, you are actually better off wearing shorts and short-sleeved shirts, in light colors—but no documented evidence exists to support this belief, as far as I am aware. You should also check for ticks throughout the day, and, upon returning home, examine yourself thoroughly and shower immediately. The shower is particularly important, because deer ticks are so tiny—perhaps the size of a pinhead—that you might miss them even if you look for them. In addition, you should use insect repellents to ward off ticks while hiking.

If you are bitten, the sooner the tick is removed, the better the chances of avoiding an illness. Try to remove the tick without leaving the mouth parts embedded in the skin. Use forceps or tweezers, or, if neither is available, use your fingers. If possible, use rubber gloves, tissues, or a piece of paper to protect your fingers from contact with the tick. If none of those is available, use a leaf (not poison ivy!). Grasp the tick as close to the skin as possible and remove it with a steady pull; try not to crush the body of the tick. Disinfect the wound and wash your hands with soap and water if at all possible.

Petroleum jelly, nail polish remover, and alcohol

will *not* cause the tick to detach. Applying a match or a cigarette is no better, and may cause the tick to explode and spread its infected contents. Do not use these methods to remove the tick; they are ineffective.

Once you have removed the tick, try to preserve it so your physician can identify it and check its infectious state. This may help in determining whether treatment should be implemented. Not every tick bite requires treatment. The chances of getting Lyme disease are considerably diminished if the tick is attached for less than 48 hours.

Insect Repellents

The easiest and most effective way to discourage insects from keeping company with you is to use an insect repellent. At one time, insect repellents containing *diethyl M toulamide*, commonly referred to as DEET, were considered the best choice. DEET has a pleasant odor, rapidly dries into a thin film, and is not oily. An application to the skin lasts six to eight hours, and an application to clothing lasts for several days. It is very effective against mosquitoes, and somewhat effective against flies, ticks, chiggers, and "no-see-ums." (My experience with its effectiveness against black flies, however, leaves much to be desired.)

Unfortunately, studies have shown that DEET is associated with toxic reactions, which increase with higher concentrations and with prolonged use. Occasional allergic reactions have been noted, as well; infants and children are more susceptible to such reactions than are adults, and some have sustained brain damage. Therefore, use DEET only when absolutely necessary to avoid being bitten alive.

DEET is available in a multitude of forms, such as sticks, cream, towelettes, liquid, and pressure spray cans. The liquid form gives you the most for your money, and very little goes a long way. Some preparations containing DEET are made especially for children. Repellents containing DEET are sold in drug stores and outdoor shops under various trade names. Look at the label before making your purchase, because the amount of DEET varies from brand to brand. Some contain 5 percent DEET, and others contain 100 percent. Avoid the two extremes: the optimum range is about 25 to 35 percent. Do not use any product containing more than 40 percent DEET, and use DEET repellents sparingly.

Another type of insect repellent contains *ethyl hexanediol*, which is safer than DEET but not as effective. It is sold under trade names such as 6-12® and Skeetogo®. Over the years, fewer and fewer products have been made with ethyl hexanediol, and it is now hard to find.

The Lyme Disease Scare

When Hugh Neil Zimmerman, the president of the New York-New Jersey Trail Conference, received a letter about a hiking club that had disbanded because of Lyme disease, he became concerned. Frightened by reports of "hundreds of cases of Lyme" in her town, the writer urged him to warn all Trail Conference members that hiking was endangering their lives. Alarmed, Zimmerman contacted Dr. Rosen, who responded:

I've come to the conclusion we are dealing with two diseases—Lyme and Hysteria. I'm quite skeptical of reports of hundreds of Lyme cases in a small town. I am connected with a hospital not far from where this person lives, which sees patients from the area. In the past two years, only seven cases of Lyme have been treated. The State Health Commission indicates that "people are being treated for Lyme who don't have Lyme"; I suspect the "hundreds of cases" fall into that category. . . .

The *New England Journal of Medicine* reports that, even in areas where the disease is endemic, the risk of infection from a tick bite is small. And an article in the *New York Times* (Jan. 4, 1994) warns that "overdiagnosis of the disease and complications from long-term antibiotic treatments may pose as great a danger to public health as the disease itself."

A hiking club disbanding because of Lyme is tantamount to motorists not driving until there is no risk of having an accident. The notion that Trail Conference members are risking their lives is a ludicrous overreaction.

Lyme disease can be serious—but if treated early, the response is excellent.

If you want to use a repellent without any harmful chemicals, try one of the alternative herbal remedies, such as Green Ban®, available in many health food stores today.[1]

Citronella, which was used before the introduction of DEET and hexanediol, is still around, and some hikers swear by Pyrinate A-200®, a preparation bought over-the-counter for the treatment of head and pubic lice. If you use Pyrinate A-200®, make certain that it does not get into your eyes, because it can burn the cornea. No research has been conducted on citronella to indicate whether it makes an effective insect repellent.

Avon's *Skin So Soft* has been highly touted as a repellent. The odor is not too bad and it is not known to be toxic. However, in my personal experience, if it works it lasts for about fifteen minutes, and then the efficacy is gone.

No repellent will prevent insects from buzzing around your head or, in the case of mosquitoes and biting flies, from penetrating your clothing. For that reason, it is necessary to treat your clothing as well as your skin, and sometimes to reapply the repellent. If

------

[1]Green Ban® has not been proven to be effective, according to Consumers' Union, and it is not registered as an insect repellent with the U.S. Environmental Protection Agency. However, some people say they have had good results with it.

you perspire excessively, you may require applications more often than once every six to eight hours.

Tips for Preventing Insect Bites and Stings

To avoid insect bites and stings while hiking, follow these suggestions:

— Don't wear brightly colored clothing or jewelry: bright colors attract stinging insects. Wear light colors such as white, light green, tan, or khaki.

— Wear long-sleeved shirts and pants if you can, and a head net, which can be purchased at any army surplus store. If you are with a work crew, wear gloves. (Some very lightweight shirts and pants are made for warm weather. Made of cotton and Supplex® nylon, they dry almost immediately and they have mesh vents to help keep you cool in hot, humid weather.)

— Avoid the use of scented soaps, lotions, shampoos, and perfumes. Don't smell like a flower. This is the only time having B.O. is an asset.

— Don't go barefoot or wear sandals during insect weather, which is from April to October.

— If you encounter buzzing bees or horrible hornets, do not swat. Retreat slowly. If retreat is impossible, lie face down and cover your head with your arms.

After a hike, take a shower or a bath to wash off whatever repellent is left. (The shower or bath may also wash off ticks, and it will give you an opportunity to conduct a tick check.)

Animal Bites

Most of us love animals, and we love looking at them and interacting with them, but they deserve our respect—and they can hurt us if we're not careful, especially when we barge into their homes unannounced. Hikers are most often concerned with snake bites and rabies.

Snake Bites

Snakes do not generally bite unless they are provoked, so when you're hiking, be aware of your surroundings and be sensitive to what's on the trail. Enjoy nature by observing it: you don't want to step on a big rattler basking quietly on a rock in the sun.

Not all snake bites require treatment. About 30 percent of the time the snake does not inject venom. When it does, the victim will recover without treatment almost all of the time. Poisonous snake bites are most serious to the very young and the very elderly. The most common poisonous snakes in the Northeast are the timber rattler and the copperhead. The rattler's bite is more serious than the bite of the copperhead.

All bites should be treated as medical emergencies until proven otherwise. If you are days away from a medical facility, it should be comforting to all members of the party, including the victim, that the odds are so favorable. If a facility is available, the decision to treat or not to treat should be made by someone skilled in evaluating snake bites.

Treating Snake Bites

Hikers are united on many issues, but the correct treatment of snake bites is not one of them. The proper first aid for treating snake bites includes these steps:

1 Immobilize the injured part of the body and, if possible, keep it at an elevation slightly below the level of the heart.

2 Keep the victim warm. This should not be too difficult since snakes are active only during the warm months of the year.

3 Wrap an Ace® bandage or its equivalent below, over, and above the site of the bite. Don't make it so tight that it cuts off the circulation, and do not remove it until you are in a medical facility.

4 Keep the victim at rest, if possible. However, if the only way to get medical help is to move the victim, then do so. Try to get to the closest road so transportation can be used if available.

5 Don't make a cross-cut incision on the bite, and don't use suction unless you know how to do it. It is estimated that about half of the people treated this way would have been better off without it. Think twice before you use the snake-bite kit.

6 If possible, kill the snake by stoning it or beating it with a long pole, but *don't endanger yourself*. Bring the dead snake to the medical facility along with the victim so it can be identified.

7 Give the victim two or three tablets of aspirin. It is a good analgesic and its use is recommended by some authorities because they believe it retards the toxic effects of the venom. Such active treatment also helps boost the victim's morale.

8 Finally, allay the victim's fears. Fewer than 1 percent of reported poisonous snake bites result in death, regardless of whether treatment is administered.[1] Many factors determine the seriousness of a bite, including the species, the size of the snake, the size of the victim, the length of time the snake's fangs are in the victim's tissue, the number

---

[1]According to the *Merck Manual*, 15th ed. (p. 2565), more than 45,000 people are bitten by snakes every year in the United States, and fewer than 8,000 cases of snake-venom poisoning are reported. Fewer than fifteen fatalities occur annually.

of bites, and the proximity of the bites to the victim's torso.

If you find the snake problem too mind-boggling to handle, you have a few alternatives: hike only in cold weather or only in Maine or Alaska, where there are no poisonous snakes. If you can afford the air fare, Hawaii is also supposedly free of poisonous snakes.

Rabies

Rabies used to be an extremely rare problem in our area, but an epidemic that began around 1990 has spread the disease from raccoons to household pets. The disease is caused by a virus in the saliva of a rabid animal. Those animals found to be rabid, in order of frequency, are skunks, foxes, cattle, dogs, bats, and cats. Rabies is rare in small, wild rodents such as squirrels, chipmunks, rats, and mice. The usual mode of transmission is by bite; rarely, the saliva may enter a break or scratch in the skin. Remember that not all rabid animals froth at the mouth and run around like mad. Avoid contact with all animals when hiking.

Treating Rabies

The treatment of rabies consists of an immediate copious flushing of the wound with water and soap, if available. It is extremely important to try to capture the biting animal. If you can't bring it back alive, bring it back dead (being careful not to damage the animal's head)—you may avoid a long series of unneeded injections. Don't bother with tourniquets; they don't do any good.

The next step is to get medical help as rapidly as possible. If treatment—namely, a series of injections—is needed for prevention, the earlier it is started the better your chances for survival. Usually your physician will consult the state health department for guidance regarding treatment. The factors considered are the species of the biting animal, the circumstances of the attack (for example, was it unprovoked?), the nature of the bite or scratch, the presence of rabies in the area, and the possibility that the animal has been immunized against rabies (such as a dog that has had rabies shots).

If the animal has rabies, you *must* get preventive treatment, because once you have the disease, nothing can be done—and rabies is nearly always fatal.

(For more information on rabies, see page 100.)

Poison Ivy

Contact with poison ivy can lead to *dermatitis venata*, a contact dermatitis caused by the rhus toxin, which is found in poison oak and poison sumac, as well as in poison ivy. A severe case can make life unbearable. The rash appears about two days after contact, accompanied by linear streaks consisting of vesicles that can be described as small blisters. It is extremely itchy and lasts for about a week or so.

Poison ivy is dangerous at all times of the year. The oily irritant that produces skin rashes and severe itching lies in canals in every part of the plant. If the canals are undamaged, a person can touch a leaf or stem without ill effects. Insects, however, may rupture them and permit the oil to reach the surface of the plant tissue. The oil may also become deposited on clothing or equipment and poison the skin later. It is stable for long periods of time, insoluble in water, and difficult to wash off.

It behooves hikers, therefore, to recognize the plant, which—fortunately—is not difficult, especially when the leaves are out. Do not look for red leaves or glossy leaves, because they are unreliable characteristics of poison ivy. The leaf structure has three features that are invariable:

— The leaves occur in groups of three, wherein the middle leaf has a short stalk and the two side leaves are joined directly to the stem.

— The leaf has smooth edges, without regularly shaped teeth.

— Each leaf is asymmetric. Often one edge is a simple, smooth curve, and the other has one or more serrations.

Once you are exposed to it, poison ivy can spread to other parts of the body, including the genitalia, via the hands. It is seen on the penis and scrotum when the toxin is transmitted in the process of urination. When I was an intern, my resident told us it is more important to wash your hands *before* you urinate rather than after. This certainly holds true if you have rhus toxin on your hands. Poison ivy is frequently seen on the face, again by hand contact. It can also be acquired from pets who have brushed up against the plant or on a trail clearing from tools that were placed in contact with poison ivy.

Even though different areas of the body may be exposed at the same time, the dermatitis can appear on other parts of the body over a period of several days. It was not spread from the original rash. It is still the result of the original insult to the skin.

If a plant contacts your skin, wash the area with soap and water as soon as possible, to remove the toxin. Scratching the rash once the toxin is washed off does not spread the disease. Soaps such as Octagon® or Kirkman's® are reportedly more effective than other soaps. If a rash develops and the itching is driving you mad, use cool tap-water compresses or diluted vinegar in a 1:30 combination with water. Burrow's solution is also helpful. Burrow's solution 1:20 can be used as a cool, wet compress for ten or fifteen minutes every hour or so to relieve the itching and loosen the crust. One Domeboro® tablet to a pint of water is an economical way of making Burrow's solution.

If these treatments do not help, try cortisone ointments such as Valisone®, Cordran®, or Synalar®. Mild cases can be treated with 1 percent hydrocortisone ointment applied three times a day; it can be purchased over-the-counter. Calamine lotion with 1 percent phenol may give relief from itching. Caladryl®, which is more expensive, may worsen the situation. One or two tablets of Benadryl® (25 milligrams), taken every six hours, may alleviate the itching.

Severe cases are best treated with prednisone, which requires a prescription. It brings the discomfort to a halt in very short order and shortens the course of the disease. With short treatment durations and low doses, prednisone can be taken safely. Longer treatment durations and higher doses, however, may cause glaucoma, adrenal insufficiency, and high blood pressure. Prednisone is contraindicated in systemic fungal infections.

Antihistamines are of little or no value in the control of itching. Jewel weed, a popular home remedy, does no good, causes no harm, and costs nothing. Prevention by desensitization, either by injection or oral preparations, has been disappointing and not without some danger.

All of the known treatments merely make the waiting period more tolerable. There are no effective immunizations, and the myth about eating the leaves to build up immunity is foolhardy and does no good.

You cannot catch poison ivy from someone else's rash. It is a self-limiting disease, and victims will get better regardless of what treatment they use . . . and even if they don't treat it at all, although that approach is recommended for masochists only!

Mountain Sickness

Acute mountain sickness (AMS) is relatively common at altitudes above 12,000 feet, but it can occur as low as 6,500 feet. The symptoms are headache, nausea, vomiting, loss of appetite, and insomnia. Other forms of altitude sickness include the following:

— **high altitude pulmonary edema** (HAPE), which can occur above 9,000 feet and is manifested by difficulty in breathing, coughing, and bloody sputum;

— **high altitude cerebral edema** (HACE), characterized by headache, mental confusion, ataxia (inability to walk a straight line), and coma; and

— **high altitude retinal hemorrhages** (HARH), which usually has no symptoms and can be seen in HAPE and HACE.

HAPE and HACE carry a high mortality rate and should be treated with great respect, if not dread.

Avoidance is the key in dealing with altitude illness. Make a slow ascent above 10,000 feet, and do not ascend more than 1,000 feet a day. In fact, some people recommend that a slow ascent be started at 5,000 feet. When my wife and I climbed Mt. Kilimanjaro, the guide kept telling us "*poli poli*," which means to "go slowly." I've been told that older people (my wife and I are considered older people) have fewer problems at high altitudes than young "jocks," who often try to ascend quickly. We went up slowly because we just couldn't move any faster—we were not capable of running up a mountain.

Most major expeditions to high altitudes now carry devices called "Gamow bags" to treat altitude illness or at least temporize until the climber can be taken down. When placed in the device, the climber is artificially "taken down" several thousand feet in a matter of minutes.

Stay well hydrated. I was advised to keep the urine "gin clear." (This is *not* meant to be a recommendation to ingest gin in an effort to stay hydrated.) If symptoms of AMS occur, take aspirin or acetaminophen for the headache. Do not take sleeping pills or sedatives. If symptoms worsen or if there is increasing difficulty in breathing or trouble with coordination,

DESCEND! If in doubt, DESCEND. A descent of 1,000 feet a day may save your life. In trekking with a group, it is important to look after each other, watching for signs and symptoms.

Medication may play a role in preventing or treating altitude illness, but it is not a substitute for *poli poli*. Acclimatization is still the best game plan. When my wife and I "went high," we used acetazolamide (Diamox®), which decreases the incidence and severity of AMS. It also reduces the incidence of periodic breathing during sleep, which is seen with AMS. If the person in the sleeping bag next to you is suffering from periodic breathing, you'll hear regular breathing and then a long, long pause (and you'll assume "this is it") before the breathing starts again.

Dexamethasone (Decadron®), a steroid, also helps to prevent and treat AMS. Recently, a drug called nifedipine was proven to prevent HAPE. All these drugs should be obtained from a physician. Remember their names if your physician is unfamiliar with AMS.

CHAPTER THREE
The International Hiker

Staying healthy while traveling is mostly a matter of common sense, so use it! My advice to the peripatetic peregrinator is: practice prophylaxis, prevent pestilence, pursue pleasure, and don't forget your passport.

Immunizations and Pre-Trip Precautions

If you are planning a trip abroad, contact your physician or health facility *now*—don't procrastinate. Inform them of your itinerary and the date you are leaving, so enough time is allowed to receive the necessary immunizations. If you have an illness or medical problem that requires ongoing care, see your physician *before departure* to make certain you have an adequate supply of medications to last the trip, and keep them in your first-aid kit—which should always be in your pack. You may require pertinent data such as x-rays, electrocardiograms, or laboratory reports for optimum care if the need arises. Your doctor may also be able to provide names of physicians or hospitals to contact in the area(s) where you will be traveling, just in case. If you don't know any doctor, contact the American Consulate, or Americans living in the area, for their recommendations. Additional information is available from the Department of Health and Human Services, which issues a booklet entitled "Health Information for International Travel." It can purchased from the Superintendent of Documents, U.S. Government Printing Office, Washington, D.C. 20402-9235; telephone number, (202) 783-3238.

Make certain you are immunized against diphtheria and tetanus. Most of us are, but a tetanus booster is required if you haven't had one in the past ten years. You also need to be protected against poliomyelitis, measles, rubella (German measles), and mumps. Immunization for cholera and yellow fever are often required, as well; check to make sure whether the places you visit require them. I know of a situation in which several Americans and a physician were quarantined in Egypt because they were not adequately immunized. For areas with a high incidence of typhus, plague, or rabies, immunization against those diseases should also be considered. Smallpox vaccine is no longer required since smallpox has been eradicated throughout the world.

Immune serum globulin is worth taking to protect you against type A hepatitis. Take this injection just before you leave because it is effective only for about four to six weeks. We now have a vaccine against hepatitis B, which is given in a series of three injections. The second injection is given one month after the initial injection and the third is given six months later. A vaccine against hepatitis A should be available in the very near future.

Pregnant travelers should be cautious about being immunized with live viruses. Make certain your physician knows that you are pregnant.

My advice to the peripatetic peregrinator is: practice prophylaxis, prevent pestilence, pursue pleasure, and don't forget your passport.

The immunizations you receive should be recorded in an International Certificate of Vaccination, which you can get from your travel agent or physician. The certificate is also available from the Government Printing Office, Washington, D.C. 20402, for a modest fee.

If the purity of the water is in question when you travel,

use boiled or chemically treated water (see pages 55–63). Don't use ice cubes or carbonated beverages. Beer is safe. If you anticipate a lot of sun exposure, use a sunscreen. If malaria is present, prophylaxis should start before you leave the United States. Your physician will outline the dosage scheme.

If you wear glasses or contact lenses, take along an extra pair, and get a copy of your prescription from your optometrist. If traveling on snow, take along sunglasses to prevent snow blindness and eye strain.

If you are allergic to any medications, wear a medical alert bracelet or neck chain. If you are using insulin, consult your physician about modifying the amounts and the time of your dosage.

Those who are going trekking in Nepal, or in any remote area, should take out evacuation insurance. If you have to be evacuated by air, you won't be able to get a helicopter unless you can guarantee payment, which is several thousand dollars. Blue Cross/Blue Shield and health maintenance organizations will not pay for this service. It would be a good idea to call your insurance company and find out what they do and do not cover.

Dr. John C. Hall offers the following practical advice for international travelers: carry with you a copy of the first and last pages of your passport, return airline ticket, traveler's checks, birth certificate, marriage license, the first page of a medical insurance policy, and any professional licenses you might have. These items would be of great benefit in the event of loss or theft.

Finally, one of the best ways to lessen jet lag is to be in good physical shape. Judicious use of sedatives while on the plane trip to modify your sleep pattern is also recommended. Sunlight can help reset your biological clock; upon arrival in a new time zone, try to spend as much time as you can outdoors.

If you are planning to travel, you might be interested in the International Association for Medical Assistance to Travelers, a nonprofit organization that provides complete health information for travelers, including immunization requirements, malaria areas, climate conditions, and so forth. For information, call them at (716) 754-4883, or write: International Association for Medical Assistance to Travelers, 417 Center St., Lewiston, NY 14092. There is no fee, but they do accept donations.

Some Frequent Travelers' Ailments
Even if you take all of the recommended precautions, you might still run into problems on the road. Some of the more troublesome ones include diarrhea, yellow fever, rabies, and polio.

Diarrhea

To quote an article in the *New England Journal of Medicine*, "travel expands the mind and loosens the bowels."[1] In another article, Dr. Herbert L. DuPont and his colleagues dealt with the treatment of traveler's diarrhea by using trimethoprim (TMP) alone or in combination with sulfamethoxazole (SMX).[2]

The combination TMP/SMX is sold under two names, Bactrim® and Septra®, and both require a prescription in the United States. In some foreign countries it can be purchased over-the-counter. Until now, its primary use was for urinary tract and middle ear infections, and occasionally for *Shigella*, which is one of the many organisms that cause diarrhea. However, the cause of diarrhea in most cases is *E. coli*, which responds to TMP/SMX. In one experiment, treated patients got well in about 30 hours, whereas victims left untreated didn't recover for about 93 hours. The drug was administered for five days, but in

---

[1] Sherwood L. Gorbach, "Traveler's Diarrhea," *New England Journal of Medicine* 307, no. 14 (September 30, 1982): 881–83.

[2] Herbert L. DuPont, et al., "Treatment of Travelers' Diarrhea with Trimethoprim/Sulfamethoxazole and with Trimethoprim Alone," *New England Journal of Medicine* 307, no. 14 (September 30, 1982): 841–44.

all probability three days would be sufficient treatment.

Be advised, however, that TMP/SMX, which is a sulfa drug, can cause a severe allergic reaction, resulting in hives and a dangerously high fever. Make sure you are not allergic to sulfa drugs before using Bactrim®—ask your doctor. If you develop a rash while taking any medication, stop taking it, and call your physician as soon as possible.

I discourage taking an antibiotic as a preventive. That has been done with Vibramycin®, TMP/SMX, and tetracycline, all of which may have side effects. However, generalized use can encourage the growth of resistant organisms, which means they won't respond to treatment. The medical authorities frown on this approach.

Pepto-Bismol® (bismuth subsalicylate) is still useful for treating the infamous "Montezuma's Revenge" (known in Mexico as *turista*). A study was done in which students attending a Mexican university who developed diarrhea were randomly treated with bismuth subsalicylate or a placebo.[1] Those receiving the bismuth subsalicylate were given either 30 ml or 60 ml every half-hour, for eight doses. The treated

---

[1] Herbert L. Dupont, et al., "Symptomatic Treatment of Diarrhea with Bismuth Subsalicylate among Students Attending a Mexican University," *Gastroenterology* 73, no. 4, Part 1 (1977): 715–18.

group did much better than the group given the placebo, and those receiving the larger doses of bismuth subsalicylate did better than those who received the lower dose.

Most of the studies involving Pepto-Bismol® used the liquid form. Since the quantities required are so large, however, it is unrealistic to carry Pepto-Bismol® if you are backpacking or are limited to 44 pounds of luggage—but it is available in tablet form. Two tablets are the equivalent of 30 ml, and my hospital pharmacist assures me that the tablets have the same pharmacological action as the liquid.

Imodium, which can be purchased over-the-counter, and Lomotil®, which requires a prescription, have been used frequently to treat diarrhea, but both of them have built-in problems, including the potential for making the situation worse. They can be used if the diarrhea is interfering with your sleep. The contraindications are high fever and blood in the stool.

The next time you go hiking or backpacking in parts of the world that are known to have a high incidence of travelers' diarrhea, have your doctor give you a prescription for ten tablets of Bactrim® DS or Septra® DS (making sure that you are not allergic to these drugs), or Cipro®, which is newer and about five times more expensive. (Cipro® should not be taken by children, nursing mothers, or anyone on theophylline for asthma.) With the onset of symptoms, take one tablet on arising and one at bedtime. The success rate is about 90 percent when the cause of the diarrhea is *E. coli*, but there is a whole string of organisms, such as *Giardia* and *Campylobacter*, that do not respond to these treatments. Therefore, it is imperative to drink and brush your teeth with safe, pure water.

Be careful of what you eat and where you eat it. When in doubt, boil or treat your water. If you do get diarrhea, drink copious quantities of liquids to replace your lost fluids. The liquids can be water, soda, tea, clear soups, Gatorade®, or a homemade solution (also used to treat sunburn), which is made as follows: mix one-half level teaspoon of salt, 2 ounces of white Karo® syrup, 8 ounces of orange juice, and 22 ounces of water. Be sure to replace as much fluid as you are losing.

Yellow Fever
If you are planning a trip to Africa or South America, be aware that yellow fever exists in parts of both of these regions. If you have a definite itinerary, consult the "Bi-Weekly Summary of Countries with Areas Infected with Quarantinable Diseases," which is available from local and state health departments. Information on known or probable infected areas is also available from the Division of Vector-Borne Viral

Diseases, Center for Infectious Diseases, Centers for Disease Control and Prevention, Fort Collins, Colorado.

If you are hiking in any of these areas, get a yellow fever vaccination. In recent years, fatal cases of yellow fever have occurred in unvaccinated tourists. Your own physician, in all probability, does not have access to the vaccine. It is usually administered at an approved Yellow Fever Vaccination Center; your physician or the local or state Department of Health can tell you where to find the center in your area. Have an International Certificate of Vaccination filled in, signed, and validated at the time of the vaccination. The immunization is good for ten years.

Consult your doctor if you are allergic to eggs or if you are pregnant before getting vaccinated. Do not take yellow fever and cholera vaccines simultaneously; allow four weeks in between—a shorter period reduces the effectiveness of both vaccines. However, simultaneous administration of immune globulin with yellow fever vaccine causes no alteration of the immunologic response to the vaccine. This is contrary to the usual practice of waiting a week or two before giving the immune globulin, which is given just before departure. This change was advocated by the Immunization Practices Advisory Committee, which advises the U.S. Public Health Service.

Rabies

Another disease to avoid is rabies, which is easier to prevent than to treat. Most countries in Asia (except Japan and Taiwan), South America, and Africa have endemic rabies, especially in dogs. According to the Centers for Disease Control and Prevention, four of the last five Americans who died of rabies were exposed to rabid dogs abroad. Dr. Ken Bernard, a CDC rabies expert, recommends post-exposure prophylaxis even if there is a record that the dog received rabies injections, because such vaccines, which have been produced in developing countries, may not provide protection. My thinking is that *all* dogs should be held suspect. The dog should be observed for ten days after a bite, even if it had the vaccine. If the dog dies before ten days, then the brain tissue should be examined for the rabies virus.

> *It is a well-established fact that if you avoid rabies, it makes for a much more pleasant trip.*

Since the incidence of rabies is low, it is usually not part of the immunization program to give pre-exposure prophylaxis. On a trekking trip to Nepal, our group was advised not to pet dogs or cats and to carry an umbrella to ward off the dogs. We were also warned that if we were bitten we had to get immediate prophylactic treatment. Since umbrellas are cheaper than vaccines, buy one.

Once the symptoms set in, rabies is nearly always fatal, so don't take it lightly. It is a well-established fact that if you avoid rabies, it makes for a much more pleasant trip.

(For more information on rabies, see page 82.)

Poliomyelitis

Wherever you are traveling—but especially if your plans include a trip to the Netherlands—make certain that you are immunized against poliomyelitis. Between September 1992 and February 1993, 68 cases were reported in the Netherlands.[1] Most, if not all, of the victims were not immunized against polio. The Centers for Disease Control in Atlanta notes that in developed countries such as Japan, Australia, New Zealand, Canada, and the countries of industrialized Europe, the risk of acquiring poliomyelitis is usually no greater than in the United States—but the same polio virus that caused the problem in the Netherlands was exported to Alberta, Canada by a carrier, so make certain that you are immunized wherever you are

---

[1]"Poliomyelitis—Netherlands, 1992," *Morbidity and Mortality Weekly Report* 41 (1992): 775–78; "Poliomyelitis Outbreak—Netherlands," *Journal of the American Medical Association* 269, no. 1 (January 6, 1993): 24.

traveling.[1] All developing countries should be considered endemic for poliomyelitis. Proof of immunization is not required for international travel. The Immunization Practices Advisory Committee, however, recommends immunization for poliomyelitis for travelers to countries where the disease is occurring.

---

[1]"Isolation of Wild Poliovirus Type 3 Among Members of a Religious Community Objecting to Vaccination—Alberta, Canada, 1993" *Journal of the American Medical Association* 269, no. 24 (June 23/30, 1993): 3104.

CHAPTER FOUR
Hiking Young and Old

The wonderful thing about hiking is that it doesn't require any special skills: as long as you can put one foot in front of the other, it has been said, you can hike. Another wonderful aspect of hiking is that it is suitable for practically all ages. From babies who can't walk yet to those well past their "three-score and ten," there are very few years in the life of a human being when hiking is not possible.

Older Hikers

> "Grow old along with me!
> The best is yet to be . . . "
> Robert Browning, RABBI BEN EZRA

When investigators from around the world convened in Washington, D.C. at the National Institute on Aging

to discuss exercise for the elderly, most of the partici-
pants at the conference had the same message: don't
overestimate the inevitability of deterioration from
aging and don't underestimate the ability of the elderly
body to respond to reasonable demands. Their conclusion was that exercise can stave off and even reverse
the ravages of age.

Exercise

Studies show that exercise can do all of the following:
postpone a decline in aerobic capacity up to twenty
years; compensate for declin-
ing central cardiovascular
function by increasing circulatory efficiency at the capillary
level; keep lungs younger;
restore the ratio of muscle to
fat in young people; and reduce sympathetic nervous system irritability.

> Inactivity has equal
> billing with smoking
> as a potent cardiac
> risk factor,
> outranking excess
> body weight, blood
> glucose, and blood
> cholesterol levels.

Exercise reverses the physi-
ologic decline associated with
aging. Dr. Ralph Paffenberger of Stanford University
Medical School, in Stanford, California, did a study of

California longshoremen and their on-the-job activity.[1] He found that the number of fatal heart attacks decreased as energy output increased. In other words, the less active workers received their rewards in heaven much sooner. Of the 3,686 longshoremen studied, those in low-energy, sedentary jobs (burning 4,750 to 8,250 k cal/week) had a 50 percent higher risk than their more active counterparts (those burning over 10,000 k cal/week); the sudden death rate was also three times higher in the low-energy group. Dr. Paffenberger concludes that inactivity has

> *Don't overestimate the inevitability of deterioration from aging and don't underestimate the ability of the elderly body to respond to reasonable demands.*

equal billing with smoking as a potent cardiac risk factor, outranking excess body weight, blood glucose, and blood cholesterol levels.

If your ambition is to become the oldest member of your hiking club, or if you are anxious for your life insurance company to make as much money on you as possible, or if you want to beat the five-score-and-ten

---

[1] Ralph S. Paffenberger, Jr. and Wayne E. Hale, "A-B Work Activity and Coronary Heart Mortality," *New England Journal of Medicine* 292 (March 13, 1975): 545–50.

record, keep hiking! However, if the spirit is willing and the flesh is weak, don't give in to the flesh. Force yourself to get going . . . start to burn calories. You don't have to be a hard-working longshoreperson to counterattack the ravages of age.

(For more information on exercise and conditioning, see pages 117–126.)

Osteoporosis

Osteoporosis is not a common hikers' disease, but it is a concern for older hikers, particularly women. I had not seen an accident resulting in a fracture on any hike or backpacking trip in which I participated until, one summer, while climbing Mt. Ararat, my wife slipped and sustained a fracture of her forearm as she approached the summit. I was shocked to witness such a casual fall resulting in a fracture. My wife's age (late 60s), race (Caucasian), build (medium), and postmenopausal state led me to assume that osteoporosis had played a role in the resulting fracture.

Osteoporosis, affecting more than 25 million people in the United States, is the most common cause of fractures in postmenopausal women and older persons in general. It results in more than 1.3 million

fractures each year, including 250,000 hip fractures.[1]
Osteoporosis can also occur in women who develop
amenorrhea (suppression or absence of menstruation),
even if they are very athletic. (In fact, amenorrhea and
athleticism are associated with one another.)

Osteoporosis is brought about by the reduction of
bone mass. Bone mass reaches a peak level at about
age 35, then slowly recedes. Throughout our lives,
new bone is deposited and existing bone is resorbed.
As we get older, resorption exceeds the deposition of
bone, putting us at a greater risk of bone fracture. At
the age of 90, for example, 32 percent of American
women and 17 percent of American men are at risk of
suffering a hip fracture.[2] And according to the National
Institutes of Health, "hip fractures occur most
frequently in people over age 65, and nearly half of all
hip fractures occur in persons over age 80."[3]

The incidence of osteoporosis increases with age,
is higher in women, affects more whites than blacks,

---

[1]Jeanne Rattenbury, "What's the Score on Osteoporosis?,"
Vegetarian Times, no. 183 (November 1992): 64–71.

[2]"Consensus Conference on Osteoporosis," *Journal of the
American Medical Association* 252, no. 6 (August 10, 1984):
799–802.

[3]Gene D. Cohen, "NIA Funds STOP/IT Clinical Trials," *The
Osteoporosis Report* 8, 1 (Spring 1992): 4.

and affects more underweight women than overweight women. Immobilization and prolonged bed rest increase bone loss, while weight-bearing exercises reduce bone mass loss. Hiking and push-ups are excellent examples of this type of exercise. Carrying a pack while hiking increases the benefit.

Calcium supplementation is one of several modalities for the prevention and treatment of osteoporosis. The usual intake of elemental calcium on an average diet is 450–550 milligrams; vegetarians get more. Studies indicate that an increase in elemental calcium to 1,000–1,500 milligrams per day, beginning well before menopause, can help to reduce the incidence of osteoporosis in postmenopausal women. I now urge my teenage patients to start taking calcium supplements. It may well prevent age-related bone loss in men, as well. I recommend taking calcium supplements until you make the obituary column or your physician tells you to stop.

The specific amount of calcium to take daily varies depending on the source and your age. The U.S. Recommended Daily Allowance (USRDA) for calcium, set by the U.S. Food and Drug Administration, is 1,000 milligrams; see Table 4.1 for recommendations from other sources.

Table 4.1
Suggested Daily Intake of Elemental Calcium

Age	NAS[a]	NIH/NOF[b]	NRC[c]
	Milligrams per Day		
0–6 mos.	400		
6–12 mos.	600		
1–10 years	800		800
Teenagers and young adults[d]	1,200		1,200
Adults[e]	800	1,000	800
Pregnant and lactating women	1,200		
Postmenopausal women not on hormone replacement therapy		1,500	

Source: National Osteoporosis Foundation, *Boning Up on Osteoporosis* (Farmington, Conn.: Univ. of Conn. Health Center, 1991).
[a]National Academy of Sciences.   [b]National Institutes of Health and National Osteoporosis Foundation.   [c]National Research Council.   [d]11–24 years, per NAS; 11–19 years, per NRC.
[e]Over age 24, per NAS; ages 19–50, per NRC.

There are a variety of calcium sources. Whole milk contains 290 milligrams of calcium per cup (8 ounces); skim milk has 302 milligrams. Eight ounces of plain, low-fat yogurt has 415 milligrams; low-fat, fruit yogurt has somewhat less.[1] Dairy products, beans, nuts, whole-grain cereals, and many leafy green vegetables also contain calcium. Broccoli, bok choy, turnip greens, mustard greens, collards, and kale are superb sources of calcium.[2]

If consuming a quart or more of milk every day is not appealing, consider calcium supplements. If you have problems with kidney stones, however, consult your physician before starting a supplemental program. Read the label carefully when you choose a supplement, and look for the percent of the USRDA, or the percent of *elemental* calcium, it contains. For example,

---

[1] National Osteoporosis Foundation, *Boning Up on Osteoporosis: A Guide to Prevention and Treatment* (Farmington, Conn.: University of Connecticut Health Center, 1991).

[2] According to a letter in the *New York Times*, rice increases the calcium absorption rate of such greens as spinach or chard (which are high in oxalic acid) when eaten with them. (When eaten alone, the calcium in spinach is not as easily absorbed as that in milk.) The letter writer, an author of books on vegetarianism, explains, "Rice neutralizes the oxalic acid in a way that other grains do not. Also, other leafy greens such as kale, collards and mustard greens have much lower oxalic acid levels naturally and are good calcium sources on their own." See Sharon K. Yntema's letter, "Rice, Too, Plays a Role in Absorbing Calcium," Letters, *New York Times*, September 29, 1993.

calcium carbonate contains 40 percent elemental calcium, so you would have to take 2,500 milligrams in order to get 100 percent of the USRDA, or 1,000 milligrams of elemental calcium.[1] Tums®, which is less expensive than vitamin supplements, contains 500 milligrams of calcium carbonate per tablet—or the equivalent of 200 milligrams of elemental calcium.

Vitamin D is required for adequate calcium absorption. Sources of vitamin D include sunshine, fatty fish, fortified milk, and fortified cereals. While vitamin D requirements increase with age, don't take more than 800 units daily—twice the recommended allowance. Vitamin D can be toxic in higher doses.

The efficacy of fluoride in reducing osteoporosis has not been established. Fluoride increases bone density, but does not protect against fractures.[2]

Smoking, as well as alcohol and caffeine consumption, aggravate bone loss, so stay away from them, too.

If you want to avoid osteoporosis and you are over 35, keep hiking; get out in the sunlight; drink milk; eat cheese, nuts, beans, whole grains, and leafy green

---

[1]National Osteoporosis Foundation, *Boning Up on Osteoporosis: A Guide to Prevention and Treatment* (Farmington, Conn.: University of Connecticut Health Center, 1991).

[2]"Fluoride and Osteoporosis," *Annual Review of Nutrition* 11 (1991): 309.

vegetables; take supplemental calcium; watch where you put your feet; and avoid menopause like the plague.

Immortality

> *"Because I could not stop Death—*
> *He kindly stopped for me—*
> *The Carriage held but just Ourselves—*
> *And Immortality."*
> —Emily Dickinson, No. 712

I once received a letter from a hiker who described himself as a life-long "health nut" who never smoked and who weighed the same as he approached his sixtieth birthday as he had at age thirty. He had been an active hiker for the same period and had climbed 14,000-footers out west.

Then he began to experience periodic pain in his left arm when climbing hills, but he continued to do fine on level ground and when going downhill. As the pain got worse, he consulted a cardiologist. His symptoms were classic for angina. At age fifty-nine, he was hospitalized for open-heart surgery and had a three-artery bypass and a mitral valve replacement.

He expressed concern to me that hikers in their fifties and sixties may be prime candidates for heart trouble. He thought an article on the subject would alert them to this ever-present danger.

Age alone is not the only factor in causing heart trouble. Other factors are arteriosclerosis (hardening of the arteries), smoking, obesity, high blood pressure, and genetic factors (strong family history of heart trouble).

There are limits to what you can do in trying to control your destiny, but you can do the following to try to achieve longevity: see a doctor as soon as you feel pain radiating down your left arm or have chest pain, pressure, tightness, or shortness of breath—with or without physical exertion—get periodic check-ups, avoid smoking, and keep your weight down. Exercise, but don't go on an ''A'' hike until you try out some excursions or easy hikes.

If you do have symptoms, let your physician work out an exercise program that gradually increases your exercise tolerance. In certain situations, medication might be required. My sponsor for the Appalachian Mountain Club (AMC) has developed angina and is still going strong. He occasionally pops a nitroglycerine tablet under his tongue if he approaches a steep climb. I do not have any cardiac problems and there are times when I have trouble keeping up with him. Angina or cardiac problems don't necessarily rule out hiking. However, if you experience chest discomfort, a change in old symptoms, faintness, or lightheadedness, see your doctor before you do anything physical.

Unfortunately, doing everything right does not guarantee life-everlasting. However, anyone with a good track record who reaches the age of fifty-nine and lives to undergo a triple bypass and a valve replacement can console himself with the thought that he would never have lasted if he smoked, was over-weight, and did not exercise. The occasional exception does not negate the fact that people in good condition tend to have fewer cardiovascular problems than their noncomplying peers. However, I have tremendous empathy for the reader who did everything right and then got clobbered. It does happen. Live as sensibly as you can and hope for the best.

Hiking with the Junior Set

Babies can be taken on hiking and camping trips at about four months of age. An aluminum frame with an infant carrier, such as a Gerry Pack®, makes life a little easier for the parents and is a necessity if you are planning more than a short trip. If no carrier is available, do what the Inuits or Eskimos do: wear a belted parka and place the baby in the space between your body and the parka. Infants usually enjoy the experience, and if the baby tends to be "colicky," the chances are excellent that the colic will disappear (at least for the trip).

Bring along a basic wardrobe plus an extra blanket, pajamas, and sweaters. For breastfed babies, food is no problem; otherwise, pack a prepared, ready-to-use formula. The unopened bottles require no refrigeration. It is not necessary to warm the formula, and nipples can be sterilized with boiling water. Bring along ready-to-eat cereals, as well as dehydrated fruits and vegetables, which can be rehydrated and mushed up. If your environmental sensitivities won't be offended, disposable diapers are extremely convenient, but they must be packed out with the rest of your trash. Improvise a contraption—by using an umbrella, for example—to provide shade on sunny days to protect the baby's tender skin. A down jacket with some pins can make a good sleeping bag. A head covering is a must to conserve body heat if the weather is cool; if the baby is perspiring, take the head covering off.

After three years of age, children can do some hiking, but they require a lot of carrying. Mom and Dad can negotiate over who gets to carry Junior and who carries the gear and food.

Older children should not be forced to do more than they want to or you will have a rebellion. Frequent rest stops with an occasional snack will grease the wheels. Consider hiking with other families whose children are about the same age as yours. A group of children usually does better than one alone.

Make certain that the children have proper foot gear and clothing consistent with the ambient temperature. Praise them to the skies for their accomplishment at the end of the hike.

If none of this appeals to you, get yourself a babysitter and have a ball.

CHAPTER FIVE
Exercise and Conditioning: The Best Medicine

The crucial factor in your ability to hike, backpack, or climb is your physical condition. A strenuous or even a moderate hike with a poorly conditioned body can be a horrendous experience for you, your group, and your leader. If you are physically fit, on the other hand, the same hike will be a breeze and you'll have a very pleasant outing.

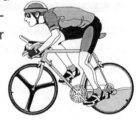

Staying in Shape

Staying in shape is a twelve-month proposition, and there are many ways to keep up an active physical fitness program. If you devote a good part of your day to earning a living, you still have opportunities to maintain and improve your shape. You can walk the twenty or thirty blocks to and from your office, for instance, instead of taking a taxi, subway, or bus; or you can walk at least part of the way. And it only requires a certain degree of mental discipline to walk up ten flights to your office and then take the elevator the remainder of the way.

Dr. Vincent Guidice advocates skipping rope as the most rewarding physical return per unit expended.

The bicycle is a very rewarding mode of transportation, both physically and economically. You can easily bike to work if it is in the five- to eight-mile range. With today's average gasoline consumption, you can probably save as much as a dollar a day. I have seen literature on folding bicycles such as the Bickerton®, which weighs 18 pounds and comes in its own carrying case. You can fly or sail to your destination, unfold your bicycle, and take off!

Dr. Vincent Guidice, who used to write a sports health column for the Bergen *Record*, advocates skipping rope as the most rewarding physical return per unit expended. You can skip rope while watching your favorite television program or listening to the radio. (The length of time that you skip rope depends on your physical condition; ask your doctor or listen to your body's signals. Exercise as often as you can without punishing your body.) All you need is a piece of clothesline rope about twelve feet long. If you want to be real fancy, you can purchase jump ropes with handles, bearings, and added weights.

More and more hikers are out all winter. Snowshoes, cross-country skis, and crampons make hiking a sport for all seasons. Dr. Pat O'Shea, an exercise physiologist at the School of Health and Physical Education at Oregon State University, tells of an incident in which a group of middle-aged men who traveled from the flatlands of Texas to Mt. Rainier scaled it easily, while many younger and more experienced climbers were unable to make it. None of the middle-aged men was a super athlete and none had any more preparation for the climb than his standard program of jogging three to five miles a day.

Dr. O'Shea has set up fitness tables that let you evaluate your own physical status (see Table 5.1). The time it takes to run 1.5 miles and your age group determine your fitness. If you are capable of achieving a rating of "good" or better, you should be able to climb a 10,000-foot peak without experiencing mountain sickness and complete the climb.

If only I practiced what I preached, I would be fifteen pounds lighter and lead only 4-D hikes!

Table 5.1
Dr. O'Shea's Fitness Table (abbreviated)

| | Minutes required to run 1.5 miles | |
Age (years)	Very poor	Good
17–29	16.3+	12.0
30–34	17.0+	12.3
35–39	17.3+	13.0
40–44	18.0+	13.3
45–49	18.3+	14.0
50+	19.0+	14.3

Source: Pat O'Shea, *The Physician and Sports Medicine.*

Conditioning the Heart

The veteran hiker who developed coronary artery disease and needed bypass surgery to improve his coronary blood flow once asked me whether his life-style—years of hiking, maintaining a healthy diet, and abstaining from tobacco and alcohol—had been worth the effort. The mere fact that he was around to send the letter following a high-risk episode can be attributed to his life-style.

The *Journal of the American Medical Association* (*JAMA*) reported on a top-notch marathon runner who developed chest pain while running.[1] A medical work-up revealed coronary artery disease, and he, too, required bypass surgery. His doctors felt that his superb condition had allowed early detection and enabled him to come through the episode with flying colors. They concluded that exercise helps most people ward off heart disease and, even though there are no guarantees, exercise should be encouraged.

Another *JAMA* article dealt with heart disease mortality in Iowa farmers.[2] An analysis of 62,000 deaths over a period of fourteen years (1964–78) among Iowan men aged 20 to 64 concluded that Iowa farm men younger than 65 years have a lower-than-expected mortality for all causes and for heart disease. That finding reflects "a life-style that includes vigorous exercise and little consumption of alcohol and to-bacco," compared with the life-styles of nonfarmers.

Dr. David F. Apple, Jr. says that smoking and exercise are incompatible, and people with low fitness

---

[1] J.B. Handler, R.W. Asay, S.E. Warren, and P.M. Shea, "Symptomatic Coronary Artery Disease in a Marathon Runner," *Journal of the American Medical Association* 248, no. 6 (August 13, 1982): 717–19.

[2] P.R. Pomrehn, R.B. Wallace, and L.F. Burmeister, "Ischemic Heart Disease Mortality in Iowa Farmers: The Influence of Life-Style," *Journal of the American Medical Association* 248, no. 9 (September 3, 1982): 1073–76.

levels are four times as likely to be smokers. Exercise lowers the cholesterol and triglyceride levels, elevates high-density lipoprotein, and lowers blood pressure and blood sugar. Dr. Apple does not claim that someone who exercises will necessarily live longer, but he does say that the quality of life is improved.

Hiking, jogging, bicycling, and canoeing are all exercises that bring about our well-being. A combination program including push-ups, tennis, and weight-lifting takes care of both the upper and lower parts of the body. It is prudent to warm up before you undertake any strenuous exercise, however, because it is important to activate and stretch the muscles that will be involved in the particular activity you choose.

Hippocrates, the father of medicine, considered walking to be the best medicine.

Recently, the American Heart Association designated physical inactivity as a fourth risk for coronary heart disease. The other three are high blood pressure, smoking, and high cholesterol levels.

The assumption "no pain, no gain" ain't necessarily so. But by "pain," I do not mean "exercise." Exercise does not have to be strenuous to be of benefit; light and moderate physical activities are beneficial, too.

Remember, the risk of developing heart trouble is five to eight times greater in inactive people with sedentary life styles. Exercise may or may not prolong your life, but it sure improves the quality. Give it a try. It's worth it.

Walking and Jogging

Hippocrates, the father of medicine, considered walking to be the best medicine. An anonymous hiker once said that he has two doctors—his left and right legs. Thomas Jefferson thought that of all exercises, walking is the best. Harry Truman and Abraham Lincoln have both been noted for their extensive walking.

Jogging was such a fad for a while that it might have lost some of its credibility, but it is an excellent exercise and gives a maximum utilization of calories per unit time. It puts tennis, bowling, chess, golf, and the like to shame. Jogging a mile in eight-and-a-half minutes burns twenty-six more calories than walking a mile in twelve minutes.

Unfortunately, not everyone can jog, for various and sundry reasons such as joint pains, sore knees, shin splints, general aches and pains, gear and equipment requirements, and so forth. Walking, on the other hand, can be done anywhere, anytime, by people of any age, and with almost any foot gear that is comfortable and offers some support. Walking and jogging are effective in combating high blood pressure and obesity, both of which contribute to the risk factor for heart attacks and strokes.

The Virtues of Walking

Aaron Sussman and Ruth Goode, in their book *The Magic of Walking* (New York: Simon & Schuster, 1967), include a chapter entitled "Why Walking is Good Medicine." In this chapter, they list the virtues of walking:

✔ A best exercise

✔ A preventive of heart and circulatory disease

✔ A first-rate weight controller

✔ A preventive and a remedy for respiratory disorders

✔ An aid to sleep

✔ An antidote to tensions, whether physical, nervous, or psychological

If you have an urge to smoke or take a midnight snack, take a walk instead . . . it is excellent preventive medicine. The President's Council says that walking, once considered too easy to be taken seriously, has gained respect as a means of improving physical fitness. Walking briskly on a regular schedule can improve the body's ability to consume oxygen during exertion, lower the heart rate at rest, lower blood pressure, increase lung and heart efficiency, and help burn excess calories. Walking is the only exercise in which the rate of participation does not decline in the middle and later years. According to the American Medical Association, walking an extra mile each day at a brisk pace will take off ten pounds a year, assuming your caloric intake remains constant.

If you decide that walking is your thing, start gradually both pace-wise and distance-wise, and work up. Try to do it for twenty minutes or more every day or at least every other day. To gain an upper-body workout as well, and to increase the aerobic benefit, walk briskly and swing your arms back and forth in a controlled motion—not flailing wildly—as you walk. Keep your arms at rib-cage level, bent at the elbows and held close to your body, with your hands in a loose fist, for optimal results. Make walking a daily and regular habit.[1] (Remember, however, that anyone who has not been physically active should get medical clearance before starting an exercise program.)

It looks as if Harry Truman, who was an avid and dedicated walker, was ahead of his time. Today's politicians might do well to follow his example!

---

[1] For more information on exercise walking, consult Gary Yanker and Kathy Burton, *Walking Medicine: The Lifetime Guide to Preventive and Therapeutic Exercise—Walking* (New York: McGraw-Hill, 1990).

INDEX

ABOUT THE AUTHOR

ALBERT P. ROSEN, M.D., F.A.A.P., received his medical degree from Downstate Medical School, State University of New York, Brooklyn, in 1943. Readers of the *Trail Walker* know "Dr. Al" through his "Health Hints" column, which he has written for the Trail Conference "since time immemorial." He has also had articles published in *Adirondac* and *Signpost*, and was a contributor to *Walking Medicine*, by Gary Yanker and Kathy Burton. Since 1978, he has been chairperson of the Appalachian Mountain Club/New York-New Jersey Chapter Safety Committee.

An avid hiker, Dr. Rosen belongs to numerous hiking clubs, including the Adirondack Mountain Club 46'ers, American Alpine Club, Catskill 3500 Club, Northeast 111, and White Mountains 4,000-Footer Club. In addition to hiking in the Adirondacks, the Canadian Rockies, the Swiss Alps, and the northeastern and western United States, he has ascended summits around the world, including Mt. Kilimanjaro (Tanzania), Mt. Montluciano (Italy), Kala Patar (Himalayas, Nepal), Mt. Ararat (Turkey), Skolio Peak (Greece, Mt. Olympus), Mt. Plavnik (Yugoslavia), Mt. Mussala (Bulgaria), and Grand Teton (Wyoming, USA).

Dr. Rosen lives in New Jersey with his wife of fifty years, Shirley, who has joined him on most of his adventures (and who, he says, often reaches the summit way ahead of him). They have a daughter, Nancy, and a son, Jonathan.